Shared Care for Neu

Shared Care for Neurology

by

Bernard Shevlin MB, ChB, MRCGP
The Surgery Team
Stoke-on-Trent
UK

Karl E Misulis MD, PhD
Neurologist, Semmes-Murphey Clinic
Clinical Professor of Neurology, Vanderbilt University
Chairman, Medicine Dept, Jackson General Hospital
Jackson, TN, USA

Martin A Samuels MD
Professor of Neurology
Harvard Medical School
Neurologist-in-Chief
Brigham and Women's Hospital
Boston, MA, USA

MARTIN
DUNITZ

First published in the United Kingdom in 2002
by Martin Dunitz Ltd, The Livery House, 7–9 Pratt Street, London NW1 0AE

Tel.: +44 (0) 20 74822202
Fax.: +44 (0) 20 72670159
E-mail: info@dunitz.co.uk
Website: http://www.dunitz.co.uk

A CIP record for this book is available from the British Library.

ISBN 1 84184 160 9

Distributed in the USA by
Fulfilment Center
Taylor & Francis
7625 Empire Drive
Florence, KY 41042, USA
Toll Free Tel.: +1 800 634 7064
E-mail: cserve@routledge_ny.com

Distributed in Canada by
Taylor & Francis
74 Rolark Drive
Scarborough, Ontario M1R 4G2, Canada
Toll Free Tel.: +1 877 226 2237
E-mail: tal_fran@istar.ca

Distributed in the rest of the world by
ITPS Limited
Cheriton House
North Way
Andover, Hampshire SP10 5BE, UK
Tel.: +44 (0)1264 332424
E-mail: reception@itps.co.uk

Composition by Scribe Design, Gillingham, Kent
Printed and bound in Malta by The Gutenberg Press Ltd

Cover illustration reprinted from
Gray's Anatomy, 38th edn, Peter Williams (ed.), 1995,
by permission of the publisher Churchill Livingstone

Contents

Preface

Neurological problems comprise a large proportion of the practice of general medicine. Common complaints such as dizziness, headache, weakness and sensory disturbances produce enormous morbidity in the general population and important neurological diseases such as stoke, Parkinson's disease, Alzheimer's disease and epilepsy afflict huge numbers of people. Despite this fact, general physicians tend to be inadequately equipped to deal with these common complaints and diseases effectively. Many healthcare professionals still labor under the misconception that nervous system problems are difficult or impossible to understand and, worse, that they are largely untreatable. This has led to therapeutic nihilism even as a new era of exciting neuroscience research has opened the doors to understanding and the treatment of many previously unapproachable problems. Parkinson's disease, stroke, headache, multiple sclerosis and epilepsy are all examples where important and effective treatments already exist. Even the most difficult neurodegenerative processes such as Alzheimer's disease and motor neuron disease are beginning to yield to the powerful tools of molecular genetics and early treatments are becoming available or appear near on the horizon.

In the face of all these advances, neurological specialists are in short supply. In the UK there are approximately 0.3 neurologists per 100,000 population. Even in the US where the number is ten times greater (about 3/100,000), there are simply not enough neurologists to provide ongoing care effectively to all the patients with neurological disease.

As the population ages this problem is bound to intensify. Furthermore it is in the patient's interest, regardless of the availability of a specialist, to be managed by a well-informed generalist who can take into consideration the complications of general medical illness and social problems, the subtleties of which are only evident in the context of an ongoing patient–doctor relationship, something which never can or should be replaced by specialists.

This book is meant to help the general physician to recognize, diagnose and manage the common neurological problems in partnership with the neurologist. Written by an English general practitioner and two American neurologists, it is meant not only to span the gap between generalist and specialist but also to provide a standard of care that can be applied on both sides of the Atlantic in an increasingly global medical community.

It is our hope that this partnership will help the large number of people who suffer with nervous system disorders receive the best state of the art care in a cost effective manner wherever they may live.

BS

KEM

MAS

Acknowledgments

The authors wish to thank Susan F. Pioli, Executive Publisher, Elsevier Science, who brought us together to work on this project; and, Alan Burgess of Martin Dunitz Ltd whose patience and vision allowed this unusual partnership to flourish.

chapter 1

History and examination

If the patient truly has a neurological problem, the purpose of the history is to discover the pace and general nature of the illness, and the examination is to demonstrate its location. More often the neurological component of the consultation is the exclusion of specific neurological disease. The approach is the same in either circumstance.

There are two basic approaches to neurological diagnosis. The first is to consider each common diagnostic possibility in turn as it presents itself during the history and examination. The second and preferable approach is to consider first the anatomic localization for the complaints. This approach ensures that uncommon conditions will not be overlooked. After a localization has been established, consideration of the possible etiologies is made.

The history

Taking the history is far and away the most important diagnostic tool in medicine, but especially so in neurology. Even an abnormal image often can only be interpreted in the light of an accurate history and examination. Yet the history is often the most time-consuming and arduous part of the whole diagnostic process. The best method of history taking is the use of a non-directed, open-ended question (e.g. Tell me about your headaches, what do you mean dizzy?). This approach works best when the patient has first complained of a new problem and had not yet developed his or her own theories about the nature of the ailment.

When time is short, a shortcut is the use of targeted questionnaires (see appendix for samples).

Why use questionnaires?

- They save time.
- They allow the patient to reflect on the problem.
- Patients will sometimes confide information to a questionnaire that would be difficult to extract from an oral history.
- Referring back to previously completed questionnaires in the patient's history can inspire insight for both doctor and patient.
- There may be medicolegal benefits; after all, what can be more robust evidence than something written by the patient himself or herself.
- They help to discover the patient's secret fears.

No matter how well we perform medically, if the patient leaves the consultation with the same fears with which he entered, the physician has failed. It is often useful to be indirect and subtle in eliciting such fears '...that may have crossed your mind or been suggested...'. The patient's preconceptions about their symptoms may also be influenced by what happened to relatives or friends who have had similar complaints. Such prejudices need to be sought or addressed.

A questionnaire is not a substitute for a history, but it certainly goes a long way on the journey to the diagnosis, often clearly pointing what one should pursue.

The completed questionnaire is best reviewed with the patient, exacting further detail and greater clarification where needed. After this exercise, it should become quite clear:

- why the patient has sought attention for the problem
- the duration, periodicity and possible severity of the condition

- the likely differential diagnosis and what examinations and/or tests will be needed to establish it/them
- the patient's expectations and secret fears about the condition.

The neurological examination

Traditionally the examination is divided into six components:

- the mental status examination
- the cranial nerves
- the motor system
- the sensory system
- tests of coordination
- the reflexes.

In general medical practice, the most common scenarios include:

Scenario 1. The patient complains of headache, dizziness or a minor head injury and the general physician wants to do a fast neurological examination to exclude unlikely neuropathology and reassure the patient.

Scenario 2. The patient may have particular neurologic-sounding symptoms, e.g., weakness or sensory disturbance or it is suspected that the patient possibly has early Parkinson's or Alzheimer's disease. In all these circumstances the exam is used to carefully make the diagnosis and rule out other neurological disease.

Scenario 3. Reports requested by insurance companies or lawyers to establish level of disability and substantiate or disprove a particular diagnosis.

Scenario 1. The basic examination

Observation

A substantial portion of the neurological exam can be performed simply by observing the patient while discussing the history. Some important elements at this stage are:

- mental status
- cranial nerves
- motor
- coordination.

Mental status integrity is revealed by listening to the patient tell the story. A patient with even incipient dementia will usually tell a disjointed story with errors in the time line and confused inter-relationships among facts. In addition, the vocabulary used by the patient can be a clue to the overall intellectual power and the magnitude of a deficit.

If, however, the patient has been brought along by someone else, usually a concerned relative who is the main history-giver, then a formal mental status examination is mandated.

If the patient himself is concerned that he may have dementia, he usually does not, but if it is the relative/caregiver who is concerned, then a real cognitive deficit is likely.

Cranial nerve examination is performed to a certain extent during the history in that the patient may be observed to have abnormal facial function, dysconjugate eye movements, and speech impediments that might indicate poor oropharyngeal muscle function (dysarthria) or language problems (aphasia).

Motor and coordination testing can begin with observing the movements and gestures of the patient during the examination. In fact, in evaluation of a patient with weakness, the ability to make spontaneous movements is an important complement to the formal assessment of strength and coordination.

If the patient walks normally and tells a coherent story, the neurological examination will rarely reveal any surprises.

Examination

Mental status

If the patient tells a good story and seems to be thinking normally, a detailed mental status examination can usually be omitted. Under these circumstances there are likely to be few surprises on formal testing of short- and long-term memory. The exception to this rule would be a patient whose chief complaint were in the realm of cognitive function, language or memory.

Cranial nerves

Olfactory nerve: Olfactory testing is unlikely to reveal pathology that cannot be deduced more easily by other means, so this is often omitted. When behavior problems suggest a possible frontal lobe disorder (e.g. changes in personality or motivation), smell should be tested as the olfactory nerve runs under the frontal lobe. In this circumstance unilateral anosima might suggest a structural problem. In Parkinson disease, loss of smell is nearly as prevalent as bradykinesia but would rarely be the sole manifestation of the disease. Tests for smell need not be elaborate. A vial with coffee will suffice for most purposes.

Optic nerve: If the patient's response to queries about recent alteration in vision is other than an emphatic 'No!', a quick Visual Acuity examination using a near vision chart with the patient's own glasses is needed. Examine the optic fundi, especially the discs. Check the visual fields by confrontation perimetry of each quadrant. Check direct and consensual pupillary reflexes.

III, IV and VI. Ocular motor nerves: If the patient complains of dizziness, check the eye movements and, if indicated from the history, carry out the Hallpike–Nylan–Barany maneuver for positional vertigo. Otherwise there is no need to test eye movements unless there are features in the history that warrant it. Positive findings in the absence of symptoms will often be inconsequential.

Other cranial nerves: Testing of the other cranial nerves can also be omitted unless symptoms point in its direction.

Motor: Motor testing can include hand grip, biceps, deltoid, and iliopsoas. Watching the patient stand on heel and toe tests distal leg muscles. This motor screen can be performed in less than a minute.

Coordination

Coordination testing is usually not necessary if there are no related complaints or if the movements on casual observation seem normal. Most coordination defects have significant symptomatic complaints.

Gait

Gait is observed as the patient enters the room, but additional testing may be needed if gait is a specific complaint. Tandem (heel–toe) is the most commonly tested stressed gait.

Reflexes

Tendon reflexes are often considered the cornerstone of the expert neurological examination, but tendon reflexes seldom show significant abnormalities when there are no other signs on examination. Nevertheless, it is advisable to test the following reflexes: biceps, triceps, brachioradialis, patellar, Achilles. The nerve root levels associated with these levels are roughly 1–2–3–4–5–6–7–8. Pretty tough to remember! To be clearer,

- Achilles = S1–S2
- Patellar = L3–L4
- Biceps = C5–C6
- Triceps = C7–C8.

Pathological reflexes looked for during a basic examination consist of a single, the plantar, reflex. After the patient's Achilles reflex has been tested, the sharp side of the hammer is used to stroke the sole of the foot to elicit movement of the hallux. Search for other pathological reflexes is not necessary unless there are other abnormalities on examination.

Scenario 2. Real concern about neurological disease

History is the real key to most neurological diagnoses. Patients seldom have neurologic deficits in the absence of complaints, which should be clearly evident from the history. Some important exceptions, however, are dementia, and depression. Although strictly speaking not a neurological diagnosis, depression is a major problem in many patients with neurological complaints.

Observation

Observation is at least as important in this second scenario as in the first. Formal examination will be cued to the complaints and observations. The components of observation will be the same as those noted above for the Basic Examination, but since the patient has a specific neurologic concern, the observation is focused on that complaint. For example, if a patient complains of tremor, the nature of the tremor is noted when reviewing the history. Is the tremor always present? Does it depend on whether the other limb is moving? Is it present at rest? With movement?

Examination

Ensure that the patient is not drowsy or inattentive because of drugs or medications; it is better that they return when able to give full cooperation to this important examination.

Mental status

Here we make an appraisal of affect (how they 'act'), mood (what our intuition tells us about what they are really feeling) and 'thought'. This last involves test of language, memory and visuo-spatial skills as outlined in Chapter 10; at any stage it may be appropriate to move on, once one is satisfied that all is normal.

Cranial nerves

A more detailed analysis of the cranial nerves including eye movements (III, IV and VI), facial sensation including corneal reflex (V), power of facial muscles (VII) and neck, shoulder and tongue movements (XI, XII).

Motor

A more detailed look at motor power, including finger abduction, hip flexion and ankle dorsiflexion. The muscles are observed for bulk tone and any spontaneous muscle activity (e.g. fasciculation).

Coordination

Finger–nose coordination and heel–shin maneuvers.

Gait

Gait testing is often performed when the patient walks into the office, but if this is not observed, it can be accomplished by having the patient walk across the room. Tandem gait is also done. The short excursion through the room is long enough, since gait disorders usually affect turning at least as much as they affect linear gait.

Scenario 3. Third-party requests

It is important to clarify exactly who wants the report and what is its purpose. The patient's account of his disability, clearly ascribed to the patient, the manner in which it is described and any supportive or discrepant findings are noted. The findings on the examination are noted objectively, but conclusions are drawn with great caution.

Examples

Example 1: History vs. examination

A 23-year-old female presents with suspected seizures. The patient does not remember these events. The family reports that the patient will suddenly fall to the floor and have shaking of all four extremities. She is drowsy and confused following these episodes.

The history strongly suggests generalized tonic-clonic seizures. However, during the examination the patient has one of her episodes while performing tandem gait. She crosses her legs and spirals slowly to the floor. The shaking is arrhythmic and independent in the limbs. During the spell, she retains the ability to respond to the examiner with eye-blinks.

The diagnosis is non-epileptic seizures.

Observation of the event was essential to the diagnosis. Otherwise, with the provided history, anticonvulsants may have been prescribed even if diagnostic tests had been normal.

Example 2: Observation during history

An elderly man is in the clinic for a routine visit, a yearly check-up.

He is judged to have Parkinson's disease even prior to examination by virtue of the following observations:

- decreased facial expression and soft voice
- stooped posture and shuffling gait when he walked
- impaired function of the hands while he is fumbling for his medication list.

Formal examination confirms the diagnosis of Parkinsonism on the basis of the following findings:

- slowness of movement (bradykinesia)
- increased tone of the arm muscles with cogwheeling
- impaired finger movements on coordination testing
- positive glabellar test (failure to inhibit the blink on repetitive tapping between the eyebrows).

Therefore, the diagnosis was made even before the examination.

Role of the GP

Establishing a diagnosis is essential. Patients can more easily adapt to a serious diagnosis than live with an unknown condition. However, there are ramifications to making a diagnosis that are not certain. For example, the diagnosis of 'high blood pressure'. Merely imparting the diagnosis to the patient might lead to more headaches and a worsening of overall perception of health. Indeed absenteeism in the two years following a vague diagnosis may increase substantially.

Often the patient needs to know the name of his illness – the so-called 'Rumpelstiltzkin effect'.

The rules are simple:

- Exclude serious pathology.
- Make the best-bet diagnosis.
- Give it the most therapeutically beneficial label and explanation.

Patient handouts can be of tremendous benefit. During a quick visit, the patient may not understand all that is said. A number of sample handouts for routine clinical practice are included in the appendix. It is important to update handouts regularly as medical information matures and to customize the handouts to be as useful as possible in a particular practice.

When to refer

Suggestions on when to refer patients for specialty consultation are included in each chapter. In general, referral is needed when:

- The diagnosis is in doubt and the differential diagnosis includes conditions for which definitive treatment exists.
- The patient is not satisfied with the expertise of the GP and wants a confirmatory opinion. This is especially warranted for conditions with poor prognoses.
- Treatment requires modalities not available to the GP.

chapter 2

Neurological localization

Basics of localization

Neurological localization is the key to neurological diagnosis. For any patient, the differential diagnosis can be narrowed substantially by arriving at an accurate localization. History and examination provide the backbone for determining the localization. This chapter summarizes the essentials of localization as they are important for clinical diagnosis.

Findings with particular lesions such as stroke, dementia, and movement disorders are discussed in respective chapters. Mass lesions such as tumors and abscess can produce damage almost anywhere in the brain, however, so an understanding of localization can help to narrow the differential diagnosis.

Dominant hemisphere function

The left hemisphere is dominant for language function in virtually all right-handed patients and about half of left-handed patients. The most important dominant-hemisphere functions for clinical practice are motor function and language.

Hemiparesis from a dominant hemisphere lesion results from fronto-central lesion. The arm and face are usually more affected than the leg, since the most common lesions are vascular. With long-standing

Table 2.1 Dominant vs. non-dominant localization

Feature	Dominant lesion	Non-dominant lesion
Language	Aphasia	Normal speech
Spatial orientation	Usually normal	Constructional apraxia
Vision	Contralateral hemianopia	Contralateral hemianopia
Calculation	Calculation errors	Calculation intact but may have comprehension and attention deficit
Strength	Contralateral hemiparesis	Contralateral hemiparesis
Neglect	Usually none	Neglect of contralateral body and space

lesions, reflexes on the involved side may be brisk and a Babinski sign present.

Aphasia is divided into a host of subtypes, but for our purposes, the important ones are:

- fluent aphasia with poor comprehension (Wenicke's aphasia)
- non-fluent aphasia with good comprehension (Broca's aphasia)
- global aphasia.

Fluent aphasia with poor comprehension is characterized by the patient being unable to comprehend language. This may not be obvious to the family or examiner, especially in incomplete cases. Patients often respond to context and visual cues, so their performance might suggest a better level of comprehension than exists. For example, if one asks a patient 'Squeeze my fingers' while the examiner holds out his hands, the patient may grasp and squeeze them, as he understands the request even without the words. It is important to give purely verbal commands, such as 'Hold up your right thumb' while giving no hint of the command by movement or gaze. It is also important to ensure that the family does not give hints.

Non-fluent aphasia with good comprehension is characterized by difficulty in speaking. The patient knows the concept he is trying to convey, but cannot translate it into spoken words. Patients with expressive aphasia are often very frustrated because they feel trapped, unable to communicate when they know very well what they want to say. When the deficit is more mild, the speech is telegraphic, with short phrases without complex construction. Word substitutions and literal paraphasic errors are common. Non-fluent aphasia is more obvious to the family and examiner than fluent aphasia.

Global aphasia refers to the combination of abnormal comprehension and non-fluent dysarthric speech. This is usually due to extensive middle cerebral artery distribution infarction.

Non-dominant hemisphere function

The so-called non-dominant hemisphere is important for spatial orientation and attention. The most common clinical findings with non-dominant hemisphere lesions are:

- left hemiparesis
- constructional apraxia
- neglect.

Hemiparesis of the side contralateral to the lesion is most prominent in the arm and face, with lesser involvement of the leg, since the most common etiology is vascular.

Constructional apraxia involves a visuo-spatial skill which is severely affected in patients with non-dominant hemisphere lesions, although dominant hemisphere lesions can produce this to a lesser extent. This is best assessed by asking the patient to draw a clock-face and set the time, or asking the patient to copy a diagram of intersecting pentagons. The person with intact function should do these tasks nearly perfectly.

Neglect is misperception of extrapersonal space. The brain contains a map of the universe which represents spatial localization. When a patient has a severe lesion of the non-dominant (usually right) hemisphere, the importance of contralateral space is reduced, sometimes to zero. Therefore, in the mind of the patient, the entire left side of space does not exist. Of course, lesser severity of lesion results in less prominent symptoms. For example, a patient with a large right hemisphere stroke may deny ownership of his paralyzed left hand when held up in front of his right visual field. On a more subtle note, a patient may deny his weakness, 'They tell me I've had a stroke, but I'm not weak' despite inability to ambulate and obvious dense hemiplegia. This denial of deficit is called anosognosia.

Left-hemisphere neglect can occur, but this is uncommon, partly because the clinical syndrome in patients with left hemisphere lesions is dominated by aphasia.

Cortical vs. subcortical localization

Diffuse and focal lesions of the brain may involve cortical tissue, subcortical tissue, or both. Table 2.2 summarizes the clinical findings

Table 2.2 Cortical vs. subcortical localization

Feature	Cortical	Subcortical
Aphasia	Common	Less common
Dementia	Common early	Common when advanced
Personality change	Common early	Common when advanced
Examples	Alzheimer's disease, Pick's disease, cortical infarctions	Multiple sclerosis, small vessel infarctions, parkinsonism

and causes of deficits with cortical and subcortical lesions. Some of the most important points to remember are:

- Cortical lesions are associated with language or visuo-spatial deficits.
- Cortical lesions are more likely to produce personality change.
- Cortical lesions are more likely to produce dementia.

Brainstem localization

Clinical findings that suggest brainstem lesions include:

- diplopia
- vertigo not due to vestibular cause
- hemiataxia without weakness
- crossed weakness or numbness – ipsilateral face and contralateral body
- dysarthria and/or dysphagia.

Details of brainstem ischemic syndromes are presented in Chapter 9. In general, causes of some important brainstem syndromes include the following:

- brainstem stroke
- multiple sclerosis
- vestibular Schwannoma.

Vestibular Schwannoma produces tinnitus and hearing loss. Vertigo can occur but is uncommon. Hemiataxia, facial pain, and facial weakness can develop from compression of the brainstem, trigeminal nerve, and facial nerve, respectively.

Multiple sclerosis produces deficits that cannot be explained by a single lesion. Diplopia with an internuclear ophthalmoplegia is common. Internuclear ophthalmoplegia is caused by a lesion of the medial longitudinal fasciculus. With lateral gaze, there is weakness of the adduction with nystagmus in the abducting eye. This is in contrast to abducens palsy, which produces weakness of abduction.

Brainstem strokes and transient ischemic attacks produce dysarthria, diplopia, ataxia, four-limb weakness and vertigo in various combinations.

Timing of deficits

Timing of the onset and progression of neurological deficits might seem to be more related to pathophysiology than localization, but the timing adds additional information to the localization to establish a diagnosis.

Onset
Onset of symptoms may be acute, subacute, or chronic. Acute deficits come on over seconds or minutes. Vascular lesions usually have an abrupt onset. The onset may be stuttering, although a gradual progression of deficit would not be expected.

Recurrence
Recurrent symptoms usually suggest vascular, demyelinating, or migrainous causes. Multiple strokes or transient ischemic attacks (TIA) in the same vascular distribution suggest that the source is in a single vessel (e.g. internal carotid). Multiple strokes or TIA in different vascular distributions suggests that emboli are coming from the heart, or alternatively that there are multiple small vessels being damaged by a vascular disease (e.g. atherosclerosis or arteriolar sclerosis caused by hypertension).

Headache
Explosive onset of headache suggests subarachnoid hemorrhage. With the first such headache, computed tomography and consideration of lumbar puncture are indicated to look for blood. Luckily, most of the time hemorrhage is not present, and this thunderclap headache is a migraine.

Migraine produces recurrent headaches which have onset over minutes to hours. Duration usually is hours.

The aura of a migraine may consist of focal numbness and/or weakness or visual symptoms. With migraine, the deficits migrate. A common complaint is numbness which starts in the fingers and ascends over 20 minutes up the arm and may then involve the face. This is usually followed by a headache. This is probably caused by a spreading depression of neuronal function across the cerebral cortex. The movement of a scintillating scotoma across the visual field in a patient with migraine is a common example of the spreading cortical depression of Lao.

Focal weakness

Acute onset but persistent hemiparesis in a young patient suggests mass lesion or multiple sclerosis. The same symptoms in an older patient suggests mass lesion or stroke. The timing is very different with these etiologies, however.

Single or recurrent episodes of weakness which progress over hours to days is most suggestive of multiple sclerosis. Progression over weeks would be more suggestive of expanding mass lesion such as tumor.

Focal weakness due to stroke has an abrupt onset, although it may be noted only upon awakening if the occlusion occurred at night. The sudden onset and localization of the lesion to a vascular territory makes the diagnosis of stroke. Occasional patients with stroke will have stuttering course, and the symptoms will fluctuate. However, these changes are stepwise rather than gradual.

Visual loss

Visual loss of sudden onset is usually vascular, with ischemic optic neuropathy being a common etiology. Rapid recovery and recurrent events essentially guarantees that the cause is ischemic.

Positive visual obscurations such as the scintillating scotomata of migraine march across the visual field, though the patient may need to be instructed to pay attention to this. Not all episodes are followed by headache, especially in the very young and very old, so the association with migraine may not be obvious in all patients.

chapter 3

Headache

Approach to the patient

Virtually everyone at sometime has a headache. The fundamental question is 'Why has this patient decided to see the doctor now?' Possible reasons for the patient presenting with the complaint of headache are:

- the headache is far worse than it has been in the past;
- headaches have increased in frequency or changed in pattern;
- other neurological symptoms accompany the headache;
- the headaches interfere with normal functioning;
- the patient has become concerned about the possibility of a serious cause for the headaches.

For example, one woman came for evaluation of typical migraine headaches. While she had suffered from occasional migraines her whole life, the recent death of a friend from aneurysmal hemorrhage raised her own concern over aneurysm. Counseling that aneurysms did not cause lifelong episodic headaches was not adequately reassuring. When MRA did indeed show an anterior communicating artery aneurysm, she could not be convinced that it was an incidental finding that was not causing her headaches.

History and examination correctly identify the cause of headache in the vast majority of patients. While brain images may make the diagnosis of tumor, sinusitis, or hemorrhage, no test can make the diagnosis of migraine, cluster, or tension headache.

Some of the important questions which should be asked are:

- How many types of headache do you have?
- What exacerbates the headache?
- What relieves the headache?
- Is there any warning before a headache?
- Are there any neurological symptoms before, during, or between headaches?

Neurological symptoms between headaches raise greater concern than neurological symptoms during or prior to a headache.

Examination of the patient with headache should include the basic screening exam plus:

- palpation of the temporal arteries (for temporal arteritis);
- funduscopic examination (for papilledema or hemorrhages);

On the basis of history and examination, the most likely diagnosis can be determined.

Differential diagnosis

Headaches can be divided into primary and secondary. Primary headaches include the following:

- Migraine without aura (common migraine)
- Migraine with aura (classic migraine)
- Cluster-like headache
- Tension type headache
- Chronic daily headache (transformed migraine; analgesic withdrawal headache)

All of these conditions can occur as secondary headaches in certain circumstances; however, they are usually primary.

Secondary headaches include:

- Brain tumor
- Aneurysm rupture
- Stroke
- Temporal arteritis
- Pseudotumor cerebri
- Brain abscess
- Meningitis

Some of the most important causes of headache will be considered after discussion of the primary headaches. Table 3.1 summarizes clinical features of some important causes of headache.

Table 3.1 Classification of headaches

Type	Features
Migraine – classic	Aura followed by throbbing, often unilateral headache. Commonly with nausea, vomiting, photophobia, phonophobia
Migraine – common	As above, but without the aura. Less commonly unilateral
Cluster	Episodes of brief unilateral periorbital pain. Duration usually less than an hour. Multiple episodes per day
Tension-type	Band-like or cranio-cervical pain. None of the associated features of migraine
Increased intracranial pressure	Pressure sensation or steady persistent pain. Visual loss or blurring is common. May have focal deficits or seizures if due to a structural lesion
Giant cell arteritis	Temporal pain with swelling and tenderness of the superficial temporal artery. Older patients

Migraine

Migraine is a clinical diagnosis. Most episodic headaches are migraine, but the symptoms which support the diagnosis include nausea/vomiting, photophobia, and phonophobia. Rarely, all of these symptoms may be the presenting sign of meningitis or subarachnoid hemorrhage, but as long as there is a recurrent history of similar headaches and there are no other stigmata of disease, alternative diagnoses are less likely.

Some general guidelines for the diagnosis of migraine are:

- If it is unilateral, it's probably migraine.
- If it throbs/pounds/pulsates, it's probably migraine.
- If there are any associated, transient neurological symptoms, it's probably migraine.
- If it comes and goes, with days free, typically lasting a few hours, it's probably migraine!

Nausea, vomiting, photophobia, and phonophobia suggest migraine. Certainly, these symptoms help to differentiate migraine headaches from tension type and sinus headaches. However, meningeal irritation from subarachnoid hemorrhage or meningitis can also produce all of these symptoms.

If the diagnosis and trigger factor situation is obvious, then forcible reassurance, a firm diagnosis, and the prescription of avoidance is the plan.

If the patient is well between attacks and there are no warning lights for serious causes of headache, then a trial of a triptan is indicated. A significant caveat here is that meningeal irritation can respond (temporarily) to triptans.

Managing the acute attack

Managing the acute attack depends on the manner of onset, severity (including disruption of activities), and therapeutic trials of available medications.

Table 3.2 summarizes the medicines used to abort migraine.

Table 3.2 Abortive agents for migraine

Generic name	Brand name	Supplied	Dose	Notes
Sumatriptan	Imigran Imitrex	Inj: 6 mg. NS 20 mg. Tab: 50, 100 mg	Start with one dose. Repeat pm in 2 hours	Use lower dose for patients on propranolol
Rizatriptan	Maxalt	Tab: 5, 10 mg. MLT 10 mg	Start with one dose. Repeat in 2 hours if needed	
Zolmitriptan	Zomig	Tab: 2.5	Start with one dose, Repeat in 2 hours if needed	
Naratriptan	Naramig	2.5 mg	Start with one dose, repeat in 4 hours if needed	Have been studies with brief daily administration for menstrual migraine
Almotriptan	Almogran	Tabs:12.5 mg	One at onset of attack, repeat in 2 hours if needed	
Prochlorperizine	Stemetil Compazine	Tab: 5 mg. Injection available 12.5 mg/ml; also available as effervescent tabs, syrup and buccal preparation	One at onset of migraine. Parenteral better for migraine	
Isometheptene and paracetamol	Midrid	Single dose: Isometheptene 65 mg, paracetamol 325 mg	Two at onset of headache, then one q1h as needed to max 5 in one day	

Triptans are the drugs-of-choice for abortive therapy in most adult patients with migraine. They have a low risk of serious side effects, high efficacy, and most importantly, they produce little or no cognitive dysfunction, thereby allowing the patient to work without being confused by a narcotic medication.

Selection of the individual triptan depends on personal preference. The most effective treatment overall is sumatriptan injection. Sumatriptan nasal spray is not far behind in speed and overall efficacy, but has an unpleasant aftertaste. Rizatriptan may be the tablet with highest overall efficacy, although the benefit is slightly less than the sumatriptan injection. Naratriptan and zolmitriptan have longer durations of action, which are particularly helpful for patients who tend to have recurrent headache.

Non-triptan drugs include acetaminophen, naproxen, ibuprofen and combination agents, usually with caffeine.

Paracetamol (acetaminophen) may be helpful for children with migraine, although it is seldom sufficient for adults. NSAIDs are often more effective, perhaps because of an additional effect on perivascular inflammation which characterizes migraine. Rectal indomethacin is particularly useful as a non-oral medication that often work faster in people with migraine because of gastric stasis, whether or not nausea is present.

Antiemetics have a powerful effect on migraine. Not only do they help the nausea but they also have an effect in reducing the vascular pain. Until the advent of the triptans, intravenous prochlorperazine was commonly used for management of refractory migraine. Even now, it is used for rescue therapy. Promethazine is commonly used by any route (i.v., i.m., p.o., p.r.).

Ergots were widely used prior to the use of triptans, and are still the only medications that help some patients. However, they sometimes worsen nausea and the addition of an anti-emetic such as cyclizine is entirely rational. Migril contains 50 mg of cyclizine in addition to the 2 mg of ergotamine; both Migril and Cafergot contain 100 mg of caffeine. Ergot preparations should not be used with 24 hours of a triptan.

Pure analgesics are commonly used, although it is best to use them only for patients with infrequent headaches. The risk of development of chronic daily headache is increased especially in patients with frequent headaches treated with analgesics.

Prophylaxis

Frequency and severity of attacks, established via a migraine diary, will dictate whether and which migraine prophylaxis to try first.

While there is not a generally agreed-upon frequency of headache that mandates preventative therapy, in general, headaches occurring four or more times per month should evoke at least an offer of a preventative agent. Patients may not want to take a daily medication to prevent a once-weekly headache, but with increasing risk of persistent headache, there should be concern over the possibility of development of chronic daily headache.

Table 3.3 summarizes features of some important preventative agents.

Beta-adrenergic blockers

Beta-blockers are frequently used for patients with frequent migraines. The risk of depression, other cognitive dysfunction, or exercise intolerance requiring discontinuation is low, but the usual contraindications to beta-blockers (e.g. asthma, Raynaud's) must be observed.

Propranolol is used for most people, although metoprolol is also effective. Nadolol may be useful as well. Patients on propranolol must be started on the 5 mg dose of rizatriptan rather than the 10 mg dose. Other beta-blockers do not require this dose reduction, and propranolol does not appreciably affect other triptans. The effect on zolmitriptan has raised some concerns, but the chance of significant alteration in bioavailability is low.

The reduction in headache frequency with beta-blockers is not dependent on the clinical evaluation of the degree of beta blockade. Therefore, cardiovascular evaluation is not generally a good guide to evaluation of headache control.

Calcium-channel blockers

Use of calcium-channel blockers for headache is somewhat controversial. Some patients with cluster-like headaches have good results

Table 3.3 Preventative agents for migraine

Generic name	Brand name	Supplied	Dose	Notes
Propranolol	Inderal	Tab: 10, 40, 80 mg	Start: 20 mg bid. Increase up to beta blockade if needed	Beta blockade not usually needed for migraine
Verapamil	Various Calan	Cap: 40 mg. Tab: 120 mg. Also slow release 120 and 240 mg	Start: 40 mg tid Max 120 mg tid	
Valproate	Depakote	Tab: 250, 500 mg	Start: 150 mg daily, increase as needed	Adjust to levels. Therapeutic levels often not needed
Cyproheptadine	Periactin	Tab: 4 mg	4 mg bid-tid	
Gabapentin	Neurontin	Cap: 100, 300, 400. Tab: 600, 800 mg	Start: 300 mg tid, max 3600 mg/d	Lower doses in elderly and with renal insufficiency

with calcium-channel blockers. Verapamil and diltiazem are predominantly used, although nifedipine has also been used.

Frequent dosing of tablets may give the best control from calcium-channel blocking drugs, but the ease of use of the sustained release formulations has made this method the most popular, not only for hypertension but also for headache.

Anti-epileptic drugs (AEDs)

AEDs are used not only for seizures but also for patients with numerous other disorders, including neuropathic pain, tremor, bipolar disorder, episodic dyscontrol disorder, and migraine. All of these disorders share at least a thread of common pathophysiology in that cyclic or periodic neuronal synchronization is involved in generation of an abnormal pattern of neuronal discharges. The AEDs may reduce the repetitive discharge of groups of neurons or potentially interfere with the neuronal loop which is responsible for the symptoms.

Details of the AEDs are presented in Chapter 8. But the AEDs which are predominantly used include:

- valproate
- gabapentin
- topiramate.

In addition, some other newer and older anticonvulsants are used, though with less solid scientific foundation. In general, the levels required to produce headache relief are lower than to produce seizure control.

Patient expectations should be realistic. No medication, including AEDs, will stop 100% of the headaches, whereas it is not unusual for AEDs to stop 100% of seizures. Therefore, a reduction in headache frequency of 50–70% may be as much of a reduction as one can reasonably expect.

Particular care should be exercised in using valproate in women of childbearing potential. The risk of birth defects is increased, particularly neural tube defects. Supplementation with folate may reduce this increased risk, but valproate should still be avoided in women of childbearing potential.

Miscellaneous agents

Chronic use of non-steroidal anti-inflammatory agents (NSAIDs) can be helpful, although there are occasional patients who will develop chronic daily headache because of these agents. In addition, there are reports of aseptic meningitis in patients receiving some NSAIDs, although this is uncommon.

Cluster-like headaches

Cluster-like headaches are far less common than migraine (migraine is more than 100 times more frequent). However, the severe distress caused by the pain, which is allegedly worse than renal stones or childbirth, can produce bizarre behavior and even suicide.

The typical long cluster headache (Horton's headache) picture is of a male (M:F = > 10:1) with an acute pain boring into one eye – 'like a red-hot poker'. The pain makes the afflicted patient pace the floor and it lasts for 30 minutes to 2 hours, recurring up to seven more times per day (usually once or twice). The 'clusters' last for up to 2 months followed by months of remission. There are often autonomic signs and symptoms affecting the painful side – lacrimation, nasal stuffiness, Horner's syndrome, but little in the way of systemic symptoms.

Acute abortive treatment

Avoid ethanol (and other vasodilators) and daytime naps – two of the most common triggers. The attack may be aborted by:

- inhaling 100% oxygen at the height of the pain;
- sumatriptan;
- sublingual ergotamine.

Pearls

- Cluster headaches are always around the eye and frontal region.
- Cluster responds well to 100% inhaled oxygen for acute treatment followed by calcium-channel blockers or lithium carbonate for chronic prevention.
- Frequent headaches of the cluster type are almost never due to serious intracranial pathology.

A commonly-used protocol for treatment of an attack of cluster headache is:

- 100% oxygen by mask
- Prednisolone (USA: prednisone) 40–60 mg daily for 5 days only
- Verapamil starting with 120 mg/day increasing by 120 mg/day to a maximum of 480 mg/day.

Sumatriptan injection is widely used for treatment of cluster, but the problem is that frequent treatment cannot be given many times per week. Therefore, sumatriptan is used predominantly to help with acute attacks when preventative therapy is being instituted or when there are only rare cluster headaches. Other triptans can be tried, although they do not have the speed of action of sumatriptan injection for acute cluster treatment.

Strong analgesics are seldom used for non-malignant pain, but some patients with cluster require opiates until longer-term definitive therapy can be effective.

Inhalation of 100% oxygen is occasionally used, although the advent of more definitive therapy does not make this as commonly used as it was previously.

In summary, cluster headaches usually occur sufficiently often and with such severity that preventative treatment is needed.

Preventative treatment

- Verapamil 120 mg b.d. increasing to 240 mg bd if needed and tolerated.
- Lithium carbonate to maximum therapeutic level (about 1 meq/l) if needed.
- Prednisolone as above reducing gradually over 3–4 weeks.

Lithium and steroids are potentially dangerous but the severity of the patient distress usually justifies such an aggressive approach.

Other cluster-like headaches

Chronic cluster headaches. In about 10% there is no remission. Treat as above.

Paroxysmal hemicrania. The attacks are shorter (10 to 30 minutes) but occur more frequently (5 to 15 times per 24 hours). It is more common in females (3:1) and responds dramatically to indomethacin, so much so that it is usually worth a therapeutic trial if the diagnosis comes to mind.

Tension-type headaches

These are the most common headaches affecting nearly 90% of the population in the episodic or chronic form. There is a continuum between tension-type headaches and migraine, in that one may lead to the other. This returns one of the first questions asked during initial evaluation: 'How many types of headache do you have?'

Diagnosis

The pain is usually described as a pressure or tightness sometimes starting in the upper neck/occiput, but often with the classical 'hat band' distribution with particular focus on the frontal region. Unlike migraine, it is non-pulsatile, mild to moderate in intensity and tends to start in the morning and worsen as the day goes on. Myographic studies have now shown that the muscle contraction theory was wrong.

Tension headaches are a clinical diagnosis. Scans and laboratory studies are usually not needed.

Treatment

Simple analgesics/NSAIDs are useful for the mild or episodic varieties, but beware of converting by overuse to chronic daily headache.

Prescribe adequate sleep – 8 hours per day for preference. The sedative, analgesic tricyclics may be particularly useful (e.g. amitriptylline) starting at 10 or 25 mg at bed time.

Any features suggestive of depression may warrant a therapeutic trial of a specific serotonin re-uptake inhibitor (SSRI) which may be used as well as the above.

Lifestyle advice is often helpful: more exercise, less ethanol, personal time and stress management. There are advocates for various other treatments, from biofeedback to various alternative therapies, but the evidence for these ancillary treatments is lacking.

Chronic daily headache

The main culprit in the production of chronic daily headache is the overuse of medications. A wide variety of medications may be involved, including simple analgesics, ergots, NSAIDs, and even triptans. Short-acting narcotics are probably the most common cause of chronic headache.

Diagnosis

The clue to diagnosis is the headache pattern, the medication-withdrawal pain often waking the patient from sleep and certainly present on waking. Abrupt analgesic withdrawal may be possible, but more often gradual tapering will be necessary while instituting the appropriate treatment of the underlying cause – often depression.

Long-acting NSAIDs may also be very helpful, even though they may occasionally be the cause.

Treatment

If one can convince patients to withdraw their analgesics, the time required for there to be relief from the daily headache can be long – from 4 to 6 weeks. During this time, institution of some sort of preventative treatment for headache is warranted, since the patients often have migraines in addition to their chronic daily headaches. In fact, the chronic use of medication was usually caused by acceleration in the self-treatment of initially-episodic headaches. The prevention may merely be institution of an antidepressant, which can help depression as well as headache, but if additional medication is needed, all of the usual preventative treatments for migraine are used.

Dangerous-to-miss causes of headache

Brain tumor

Brain tumors are responsible for a very small proportion of patients with headache. The headache usually has the following features:

- continuous;
- most prominent in the morning;
- associated with other neurologic symptoms and/or signs.

Only a small minority of patients with brain tumors have no other findings. Common findings include:

- focal weakness and/or numbness;
- seizures;
- papilledema;
- confusion or personality change.

When all of these features are absent, the risk of brain tumor is very low.

Emergent diagnosis of brain tumor is seldom needed, since for most, early diagnosis does not significantly alter treatment or outcome. Diagnosis is made by imaging. A mass lesion is seen on the MRI or CT scan.

The relationship between brain tumor and headache

- Brain tumors are relatively uncommon; the average family doctor will only see about 5 or 6 in his or her entire career.
- Only about half of brain tumor patients have headache at presentation.
- Other symptoms or signs are likely to override the headache at presentation. For example, late onset epilepsy, neurological findings, previous cancer (lung, breast) are often present.
- Early diagnosis is unimportant in many brain tumors. They may be so fast-growing (e.g. glioblastoma multiforme, the most common primary brain tumor) as to be rapidly fatal, or so slow-growing (e.g. most meningiomas) that a few weeks or even months of delay in diagnosis will not affect outcome.
- This leaves less than one brain tumor per medical lifetime where one may hurt the patient by not getting it right.

How not-to-miss the tumor that counts

- Although brain tumor headaches are not all caused by raised intracranial pressure, suggestive features in the history mandate further tests. Viz. headache on waking, nausea and vomiting, worse on coughing/sneezing, or other Valsalva maneuvers.
- Since over 80% of us have headaches, the patient with the brain tumor is likely to have had a headache in the past. Therefore watch for the change in headache severity, quality, pattern, or location.
- Always do the quick neurological examination.
- In children, listen to the parents. They are experts at picking up the subtle changes in the child which may be the tumor's presenting feature.

Aneurysmal hemorrhage

The typical presentation of aneurysmal hemorrhage consists of the acute onset of a headache, maximal at the onset. The onset is very acute, often described as an exploding or thunderclap headache. Onset can be at rest but often happens during exertion such as sports or stress. Neck pain may develop within the first few hours after onset. The duration is usually measured in days to weeks. A headache that spontaneously resolves after minutes to hours is usually not due to an aneurysmal hemorrhage.

Intracranial aneurysms are responsible for a very small proportion of headaches. When a patient presents with the acute onset of the thunderclap headache, CT followed by LP (if the CT is normal) is usually needed, even if there is a previous history of migraine. Nevertheless, these studies are usually normal. Clinical findings which are more worrisome for aneurysm are:

- abrupt onset of headache (maximal at the onset);
- alteration of consciousness at onset;
- diplopia;
- persistence of the headache for days.

Alteration of consciousness is uncommon in patients with migraine, although young women with basilar migraine or patients with hemiplegic migraine may develop alteration of consciousness. When this develops, extensive investigation for intracranial catastrophe should be entertained.

Unfortunately, there are no clearly dependable findings on history or examination that definitively differentiate between subarachnoid hemorrhage and migraine. As mentioned already, response to triptan treatment cannot distinguish between these possibilities.

Acute frontal sinusitis

Acute tenderness over a frontal sinus with symptoms or signs of infection may herald imminent rupture of the thin posterior sinus wall into the brain; urgent referral is mandated. X-rays can suggest sinusitis. CT of the sinuses best shows the status of the sinuses. MRI often exaggerates findings of sinusitis.

Giant cell arteritis (Temporal arteritis)

Giant cell arteritis is an uncommon cause of headache, but should be considered in almost every elderly patient who presents with a new or changing headache. While physicians are usually quite good about correctly diagnosing primary headaches, giant cell arteritis can be overlooked. Often the history is of severe headache which may have a temporal predominance, but may not be identified as localized particularly in the temporal region. Classic features include:

- temporal headache
- temporal artery which is prominent and tender, and
- elevated erythrocyte sedimentation rate (ESR).

When a patient has no prior history of headache, the diagnosis is easier, but the first potential pitfall in diagnosing this condition is when there is a long history of headache. Unless the details of the history are obtained, a change in character may not be appreciated. Also, the headache may not be localized around the temporal arteries by the patient, and in fact the pain may extend through the side of the head and down into the neck. Checking the ESR should be routine in an elderly patient with new or changing headache, but the ESR is not elevated in all patients. Even temporal artery biopsy may not be definitive, since the inflammation is segmental. Therefore, temporal artery biopsy is not mandatory for most patients, and a typical clinical presentation supported by an elevated ESR warrants treatment. The risk of treatment when not necessary is eclipsed by the potential for blindness or stroke if the diagnosis is not made.

The treatment is prednisolone 40–60 mg/day for one month followed by a slow tapering of about 10% of the starting dose per week, assuming clinical evaluation and ESR measurement have shown improvement in the disease. If the patient develops signs or symptoms of ocular or brain ischemia, immediate treatment with high-dose parenteral steroids is warranted (i.e. about 1 g of methylprednisolone intravenously per day for 7–10 days).

Subdural hematoma

The brain shrinkage that occurs in the elderly means that even minor trauma can trigger a subdural hemorrhage. Indeed only about half of patients with proved subdural hematomas give a history of trauma retrospectively. Treatment with anticoagulants greatly increases the incidence of intracranial bleeding after otherwise insignificant head injury. Watch for fluctuating symptoms – fluctuating headache (> 75% have headache) and fluctuating level of consciousness. If there is any suggestion of intracranial bleeding an urgent brain image (CT or MRI) is needed.

Cerebral abscess

Cerebral abcess usually presents with progressive severe headache with markers for infection (fever, raised white cell count). Most patients with cerebral abscess have other signs of neurological dysfunction, such as lethargy or confusion, seizures, or focal neurological deficits.

Diagnosis is made on the basis of a brain image (CT or MRI) that shows an enhancing lesion. Unfortunately, MRI and CT are not able to definitively distinguish between tumor and abscess. Therefore, biopsy or excision may be needed. Referral to a neurosurgeon is made in all patients with cerebral mass lesions, but the referral should be urgent if there is reasonable possibility that the lesion could be an abscess.

Meningitis

Meningitis produces headache associated with nausea and photophobia that can resemble a migraine, and can also resemble subarachnoid hemorrhage. Neck pain is common in meningitis and subarachnoid hemorrhage, although it can occasionally occur in patients with migraine, usually as a secondary muscle contraction from the pain.

Diagnosis is made by lumbar puncture (LP). If the patient has any symptoms which suggest focal or generalized brain dysfunction, a brain image (CT or MRI) should be done prior to the LP, in case there is significant cerebral mass effect. While waiting for the image to be obtained, antibiotics often should be given prior to the LP. While this is not optimal, the potential delay in treatment can be life-threatening.

Pseudotumor cerebri

Benign intracranial hypertension is another term for pseudotumor cerebri, where there are the signs and symptoms of increased intracranial pressure without mass lesion or hydrocephalus. This is seen mainly in young obese females, although this is not invariable. Papilledema is the main finding on examination, and other objective neurological signs raise doubt about the diagnosis.

Diagnosis is suspected by papilledema without other findings on exam in a young person, especially an obese female. Confirmation is made by CT or MRI scan plus LP. The scan is either normal or shows slit-like ventricles. LP shows increased opening pressure. Otherwise, the CSF analysis is normal, although protein levels may be low.

Pearls
- Addressing the patient's fears is essential.
- The neurological examination should pick up any warning signs.
- Steroids will relieve virtually any headache within a few hours.
- Unilateral headaches (unless cluster) often respond to indomethacin.
- Episodic headaches are almost always benign.
- Ask about how many different types of headaches the patient has. Classification can then be much easier.
- Headaches that respond to triptans are not necessarily migraine.
- Think about temporal arteritis in the elderly patient with new or changed headache.

When to refer

- Neurological deficit.
- Refractory headache.
- Inadequate doctor–patient relationship for the long haul.
- Trust your intuition; if something doesn't feel right, get a second opinion.
- Positive neurological signs usually mandate imaging.

chapter 4

Dizziness

'Dizziness' is not a medical term. When patients use words such as constipation, angina or migraine there is a certain definite commonality of language and understanding between patient and doctor. However, 'dizziness' is an attempt to label an experience for which they have an inadequate vocabulary and usually no shared reference experience. As such 'dizziness' is used interchangeably, contingent upon region and culture, with 'giddiness', 'having a funny turn', 'coming over queer', 'going mazey' and many others. The declaration of 'vertigo' usually, but not always, implies a sense of rotation.

Approach to the patient with dizziness

The first fact to discover is what precisely the patient means by the term. Sometimes the open-ended invitation to describe the symptom can deliver useful information, but here patience is the order of the day. 'Let the patient talk for long enough and he will tell you the diagnosis' is never more true than here. Sadly such a strategy will often tax one's patience, and the patience of those in the full waiting room. The questionnaire can save an enormous amount of time here, especially if prefaced by the doctor's insistence that he or she needs a precise description of the patient's sensory experience.

After evaluating the questionnaire and clarifying the patient's description, we should be in a good position to classify the complaint as:

- True vertigo – with a perception of movement
- Near-syncope or pre-syncope (the sensation of impending faint)
- Psychological – anxiety, panic attacks and some subtypes of depression
- Sensory deficit syndromes – uncertainties of body and limb position
- Ataxia

Common causes of vertigo are shown in Table 4.1. Treatments are presented in Table 4.2.

Examination of the patient being evaluated for dizziness should consist of the basic screening exam plus special attention to the following:

- hearing
- eye movements
- gait
- facial movements
- speech
- blood pressure with changes in position
- Hallpike (Nylen–Barany) maneuver.

Table 4.1 Causes of vertigo

Peripheral	Central	Systemic
Vestibulopathy	Brainstem ischemia	Hypothyroidism
Benign positional vertigo	Brainstem tumors	Diabetes mellitus
Meniere's disease	Multiple sclerosis	Drugs
Post-stapedectomy	Vascular malformations	Hypotension
Cholesteatoma	Migraine	Vasculitis
Post-traumatic	Seizures	Anemia
	Spinocerebellar degenerations	Infections

Table 4.2 Treatment of vertigo

Generic name	Brand name	Supplied	Dose	Notes
Betahistine	Serc	Tabs: 8, 16 mg	Start 16 mg tid, maintenance 24–48 mg/day	
Cyclizine	Valoid	Tab: 50 mg	50 mg tid	Available as i.v. and i.m.
Promethazine	Avomine Phenergan	Tab: 25 mg Tab: 25, 10 mg; also liquid (elixir) 5 mg/5 ml	1–2 prn, max 4/day	
Diazepam	Generic diazepam	Tab: 2, 5, 10 mg; also oral solution 2 mg/5 ml, 5 mg/5 ml	Start: 2 mg tid, max 10 mg tid	Available as i.v. and i.m.
Lorazepam	Ativan	Tabs: 1, 2.5 mg	Start: 0.5 mg tid, max 2 mg tid every 72 hours	Available as i.v. and i.m.
Scopolamine	Scopoderm	Patch: 1.5 mg	1 patch changed every three days	

Hearing

Attention to the patient during the history will reveal any major hearing defect.

Eye movements

The patient's eyes track the examiner's finger looking for nystagmus and inquiring about diplopia.

Tip: don't have the patient follow the finger too far laterally, as some normal patients will show nystagmus, which is normal (end point nystagmus).

Gait and limb coordination

In a very acute case, with the patient hanging on for dear life, gait and balance testing are impossible and unnecessary, though simple upper limb coordination testing is appropriate. In the more subtle or between-episode cases, walking and turning, the more demanding heel–toe walking, Rombergism and finger–nose testing will be either re-assuringly normal or alert one as to persisting problems.

Facial movement and speech

This is usually assessed during history-taking and seldom requires specific testing.

Blood pressure

Reports of dizziness when the patient stands should raise concern over orthostatic hypotension. Patients may usually complain of light-headed or some other lay-counterpart of presyncope when they stand. On the other hand, others may report imbalance or a vague dizziness without a clear presyncope.

Factors which may predispose to orthostatic hypotension include:

- diabetes
- peripheral neuropathy
- Parkinson's disease and related parkinsonian disorders.

Hallpike maneuver

In addition, the Hallpike (Nylen–Barany) maneuver is commonly performed in patients with true vertigo. The patient is seated with head straight then abruptly laid back on the table so that the head is hanging 30 degrees below the horizontal. After observing for nystagmus, the patient is then sat upright and the maneuver repeated twice more, one with the head being turned to the left 45 degrees while down and the other turned 45 degrees right while down. The nystagmus in benign positional vertigo is typically with the fast phase towards the lower ear. Differentiation of central from peripheral vertigo is the key to this maneuver.

Limb ataxia

Gait ataxia does not necessarily indicate a central lesion, but limb ataxia does, as individual movements of the limbs do not depend on the vestibular system for feedback. Symptoms include:

- diplopia
- visual loss
- disturbance of consciousness, or
- focal weakness.

In the absence of any of these findings, the chance of serious causes of true vertigo is very low.

Diagnosis of vertigo

Peripheral causes of vertigo are suggested by the following findings on the Hallpike maneuver:

- latency of 5–10 s to onset of nystagmus and vertigo;
- duration of nystagmus of less then one minute;
- fatigability of the response to successive maneuvers;
- direction of the nystagmus towards the lower ear;
- intensity is severe.

Central vertigo is suggested by:

- immediate onset of nystagmus and vertigo;

- persistent symptoms beyond that seen with peripheral lesions;
- no fatigability with successive maneuvers;
- inconsistent or complex direction(s) of movement during the nystagmus;
- intensity often mild to moderate, less severe than with peripheral causes.

Remember!

True vertigo is characterized by a sense of rotation. Some patients feel they are moving within the room, whereas others feel the room is moving around them. There is no significance to this perceptive distinction. True vertigo is usually benign, and peripheral in origin, with vestibulopathy being the most common cause. Peripheral vertigo is often associated with gait difficulty but with no other symptoms or signs of neurological disturbance.

Therefore, **Beware!**

Neurological causes of vertigo

Among the serious neurological causes of true vertigo are:

- brainstem stroke – infarction or hemorrhage;
- multiple sclerosis;
- tumors in the brainstem region and cerebello-pontine angle;
- basilar migraine;

Brainstem stroke and transient ischemic attacks (TIA) are almost always associated with findings other than vertigo and ataxia, with the most common being diplopia, appendicular ataxia, dysarthria, and focal face and/or limb weakness. Brief episodes of isolated vertigo may be due to brainstem TIA, presumably because the regional ischemia was insufficient to produce other symptoms.

Internal auditory artery infarction is an uncommon cause of vertigo. Unlike most ischemic disease which is most prominent in the elderly, internal auditory artery infarction tends to occur in younger patients, especially in association with lupus, polyarteritis nodosa, or syphilis.

Multiple sclerosis can produce almost any neurological symptoms and sign, but isolated vertigo is unusual. Nevertheless, one should always ask a patient with unexplained vertigo about not only previous attacks of vertigo but also other attacks which might have been demyelinating, including visual loss (optic neuritis), leg weakness (transverse myelitis), or hemiparesis.

Tumors in the posterior fossa are most common in children but can occur at any age. Midline tumors such as medulloblastoma usually produce ataxia, nausea, and vomiting rather than vertigo. Infiltrating gliomas of the brainstem and ependymomas, also tend to present with headache, nausea, and ataxia. Vestibular Schwanomma (often incorrectly called acoustic neuroma) may produce vertigo but this is usually a late finding. Tinnitus and hearing loss are the early symptoms.

Migraine is associated with vertigo more often than would be expected by chance. This is not only basilar migraine but also more typical migraine in adults. Basilar migraine is an uncommon disorder usually of teens, with severe occipital headache. Visual aura is common, and is followed by numbness and tingling of the lips, hands, and feet. These symptoms are usually bilateral. Ataxia and dysarthria follow and may lead into confusion or loss of consciousness. Vertigo may occur in this symptom complex, but is overshadowed by the other symptoms.

Otologic causes of vertigo

Important otological causes include:

- vestibulopathy
- Meniere's disease
- benign positional vertigo
- ruptured round window
- post-stapedectomy
- cholesteatoma.

The latter three are extremely rare, but need to be considered in a new acute case of vertigo. Vestibulopathy, Meniere's disease, and benign positional vertigo are discussed later in this chapter.

Ruptured round window is usually from barotrauma, rarely from exertion. Onset of the symptoms is usually dramatic and with tinnitus.

Post-stapedectomy. Occasional patients who have had stapedectomy will develop vertigo or even more severe neurological complications including meningitis. It may occur as a late complication many years after surgery and is usually accompanied by reduced hearing and tinnitus.

Cholesteatoma is usually characterized by a history of persistent foul aural discharge and otoscopic examination may reveal the attic abnormality. A specialist examination is needed. The onset of vertigo is a worrying feature, heralding as it does, that the progressive enlargement of the mass is eroding into the semicircular ducts. Alteration of pressure in the external auditory canal, by sealing it with the tragus and exerting gentle pressure, may produce the acute vertigo, proving this to be the case, and mandating urgent referral to avert the disaster of intracranial infection.

Vestibulopathy

Vestibulopathy encompasses the clinical syndromes of labyrinthitis and vestibular neuronitis. The presence of the latter as a distinct pathophysiological entity is debatable. Therefore, the term vestibulopathy is preferred. The cause is unknown for most patients, and may have multiple potential causes. Infections and allergies have been implicated without solid evidence.

Patients present with single or recurrent episodes of vertigo which is exacerbated by head movement. Patients may occasionally feel light-headed in association with this, but frank neurological symptoms and signs are absent.

Benign positional vertigo

Benign paroxysmal positional vertigo (BPPV) is sometimes called

Barany's disease. This is vertigo which is typically associated with certain head positions. The patient suffers episodes of vertigo often with nausea and vomiting. Duration of the episodes is less than one minute. These episodes tend to be lessened late in the day and are minimized by keeping the head still in a position which does not provoke the vertigo.

Position change can exacerbate almost any cause of vertigo, even brainstem ischemia or multiple sclerosis. Therefore, a positional character does not make the diagnosis of BPPV.

Meniere's disease

Meniere's disease may be due to excess endolymphatic fluid in the semicircular canals or may be a recurrent immune mediated disorder in which there are circulating antibodies directed against components of the inner ear. Patients present with:

- severe vertigo;
- nausea and vomiting;
- fluctuating hearing loss;
- often vague pressure sensation in the ear.

The hallmark of the diagnosis is the episodic nature of the attack, leaving the patient 'normal' after the first, but later causing progressive cochlear damage.

The underlying cause is unknown for most patients, although there are a number of potential causes, including autoimmune disease and bacterial or viral infections.

There are a wide variety of antihistamines, antiemetics, and sedatives which are helpful. Benzodiazepines are especially effective since they aid both the vertigo and the accompanying anxiety. Long-term management consists of:

- low-salt diet
- diuretics
- anti-histaminic agents.

Betahistine is the first-line treatment. Corticosteroids are used in some patients with bilateral symptoms, especially if the pathophysiology is thought to be autoimmune.

Drug effects

As much as 10% of dizziness is drug-related. Always check the medications. Some common classes of drugs which can produce vertigo (or other dizziness) are:

- anticonvulsants
- any psychotropic
- some antihypertensives
- analgesics.

Syncope and pre-syncope

The final common pathway to syncope is decreased perfusion of the brain. Important causes are:

- Orthostasis
- Subclavian steal
- Extracranial carotid or vertebral stenosis
- Hypovolemia
- Arrhythmia
- Hypotension

Orthostasis can occur in the setting of associated disorders, often with autonomic neuropathy.

- Idiopathic orthostatic hypotension
- Parkinson's disease
- Multiple system atrophy
- Diabetic neuropathy

As with other causes of hypotension, the key to diagnosis is the absence of symptoms of CNS damage.

Other causes of orthostatic hypotension include:

- Acute blood loss (beware occult blood loss as in ruptured ectopic pregnancy, undeclared gastrointestinal bleeding)
- Myocardial ischemia (beware the silent MI of the diabetic, the elderly and previous cardiac surgery)
- Aortic stenosis. Mitral valve disease and hypertrophic obstructive cardiomyopathy (HOCM) of young adults can also present like this)

Psychological causes

The questionnaire will reveal the additional tell-tale symptoms of psychological distress and the patient's secret fears. The examination proceeds with particular gravitas with the additional objective of addressing and these secret fears.

Depression, especially the agitated depression, can have 'dizziness' as part of the presenting symptom-complex. If in doubt, the depressing effect of a depressed patient often triggers the experienced physician's concern.

Anxiety. The general physician can often make a definitive diagnosis, knowing as he or she does the patient's background history, life stresses, family history and psychological stressors.

Panic attacks can sound initially very 'organic' with predominance of physical symptoms – palpitations, breathlessness, sweating, but the time-scale may be very helpful in teasing out the diagnosis. The 'dizziness' here is usually from hyperventilation and the feeling of being cut off from reality – 'de-realization'.

Exclusion of both pathology and the patient's fears with a well-conducted physical examination is essential. If further tests are needed to settle either, they are invariably cost-effective.

Sensory deficit syndromes

Imbalance is one potential medical symptom which may present with the clinical complaint of 'dizziness'. Ataxia is a diagnostic term imposed after neurological examination, it is not a chief complaint. Some important causes of imbalance are:

- peripheral neuropathy
- alcoholism
- stroke
- Parkinson's disease
- age (multi-sensory deficit syndrome)

These and other disorders affect balance in one of the following ways:

- defective signal processing in the brain and/or spinal cord;
- defective sensory input;
- defective execution of planned movements.

The sensory inputs which the brain needs for balance are: proprioceptive, vestibular, and visual. Any one of these may be absent with only mild deterioration in function, but loss of more than one of these modalities may be associated with prominent imbalance.

Peripheral neuropathy

Peripheral neuropathy produces imbalance by loss of the normal position sense in the feet. Position sense is just one of the signals which allows one to know which direction joints are moving. Only a small subset of patients will describe the resulting imbalance as 'dizziness'. However, the elderly will often fail to ascribe part of their imbalance to sensory loss, perhaps because they consider some sensory loss to be a normal part of aging.

Diagnosis of neuropathy can be made by sensory testing; that is:

- sharp-dull differentiation;
- proximal vs. distal sharp sensation;
- vibration sensation;
- proprioception.

These sensory tests are not routinely performed on patients; however, they should be performed if ankle reflexes are absent or if symptoms suggest a sensory-deficit syndrome.

Alcoholism

Chronic ethanol abuse may result in degeneration of the cerebellar vermis. This impairs gait and stance while sparing the upper limbs and speech; peripheral neuropathy as above may compound the symptoms and signs.

The history, examination and hematological and biochemical markers for alcohol excess establish the diagnosis and an MRI will show the classic appearance of superior midline vermian atrophy on the midline sagittal images.

Treatment consists of nutritional supplementation including multi-vitamins. Cessation of intake of ethanol is essential. Unfortunately, despite the success of this treatment, the ataxia can remain quite disabling.

Alcoholism can produce cerebellar ataxia which spares limb movements. This degeneration of the cerebellar vermis has a typical appearance on autopsy and sagittal MRI images. This development is most common in individuals who have neglected their nutrition while imbibing large amounts of ethanol. Diagnosis is established by investigation for cerebellar masses and infarcts with imaging, and search for metabolic causes of ataxia in a patient with a typical history of ethanol excess.

Stroke

Stroke seldom produces imbalance in the absence of other signs of neurological dysfunction. Most patients with gait ataxia have: limb ataxia, diplopia, dysarthria, dysphagia, and/or focal weakness. Therefore, during examination of a patient with imbalance, examination of limb function and other brainstem functions is essential.

Parkinsonism

Parkinsonism is discussed in further detail in Chapter 7. Briefly, Parkinsonism can be due to Parkinson's disease, stroke, drugs, head injury, or one of a number of degenerative diseases for which Parkinson's-like symptoms are just one clinical component. Parkinsonism is associated with imbalance which usually manifests as frequent falling. Corrective reflexes are impaired. This results in an imbalance which is not just merely due to the slowness of movement which is also a characteristic of this disorder.

The diagnosis of Parkinsonism is based on a constellation of findings including imbalance, slowness and paucity of movement, and tremor.

Among the disorders which can resemble Parkinsonism, frontal lobe structural lesions (stroke, tumor) and normal-pressure hydrocephalus are the most important. Therefore, while a clinical diagnosis of Parkinsonism may seem definitive, some sort of brain image is often warranted.

Age

Aging patients frequently have progressive deterioration in balance. In most patients this is not due to a single pathological condition but rather secondary to the multiple slings and arrows of life. Among the

Pearls

- Loss of consciousness is never due to a peripheral vestibular disorder.
- Acute vertigo of peripheral origin is virtually always accompanied by nystagmus.
- Gait ataxia is seen in peripheral causes of vertigo; limb ataxia is not.
- Syncope is not due to carotid vascular disease, but it may be seen with basilar disease.
- Central causes of vertigo almost always have associated neurological findings.
- Vertigo without tinnitus or hearing loss is almost never due to vestibular Schwannoma.
- Always consider concurrent medicines in a patient presenting with dizziness.

contributing factors are deterioration in vision, cervical spondylosis, loss of vestibular function, and perhaps some neuropathy which affects position sense. Not all senior citizens with ataxia have Parkinsonism, although this is a common disorder

When to refer

- *ENT.* Otological emergencies. Suspected perilymph leak (ruptured round/oval window), advancing cholesteatoma.
- *Cardiology.* Cardiac cause presenting as syncope and pre-syncope (silent MI, exercise syncope; suspected arrhythmia)
- *Medical admission.* Suspected occult gastrointestinal hemorrhage; pulmonary embolism
- *Neurology.* Cerebrovascular disease, sensory deficit syndromes, demyelinating disease such as multiple sclerosis; neuro-degenerative diseases.

chapter 5

Weakness and fatigue

Approach to the patient

The differential diagnosis of weakness and fatigue is as broad as that of dizziness. These are non-specific complaints that can have a multitude of specific causes. Among these complaints is 'Tired-all-the-time' or TATT. As with all complaints, the first task is to correctly classify the problem. The general classification of disorders, which are commonly diagnosed, includes:

- diffuse muscle weakness
- focal muscle weakness
- lack of initiative with intact strength.

Diffuse muscle weakness can be due to neuromuscular disease, hypothyroidism or other metabolic disorder. Focal muscle weakness can be of CNS or PNS origin, and detailed examination can usually correctly localize the lesion. Lack of initiative can be due to metabolic disorder such as diabetes, thyroid disorder, but this is more commonly due to depression or chronic illness. These conditions will be covered in turn (Table 5.1).

Neurological causes of weakness

Usually the patient will quickly declare which areas of the body are affected. Even the generalized weaknesses have an organic feel to the way they are presented.

History should concentrate on all of the cardinal features of any historical description. How long, how often, what makes it worse, what makes it better, etc? However, some special questions should be asked to clarify the diagnosis.

- Where are you weak? What part(s) of your body?
- Did anything cause the weakness/fatigue, or was there any significant life-event at the onset?
- Are there any sensory symptoms? Numbness? Dysesthesias? Pain?

Some brief examples from history, alone:

- Generalized weakness and muscle pain which occurred after a night of binge drinking suggests alcoholic rhabdomyolysis.
- Gradual onset of weakness in the intrinsic muscles of the hand with numbness in mainly the little finger suggests ulnar neuropathy, with the most common cause being compression at the elbow.
- Progressive weakness with no sensory symptoms with muscle twitching suggests motoneuron diseases such as amyotrophic lateral sclerosis (ALS).

Diffuse weakness

Diffuse weakness is divided as follows:

- Is the problem weakness or fatigability?
- Is there weakness of muscles supplied by the brainstem – dysarthria, dysphagia, diplopia, facial weakness?
- Are there sensory symptoms?

Diffuse weakness with cranial nerve involvement is usually due to neuromuscular disorder. ALS (a form of motorneuron disease) presents with weakness with fasciculation and often muscle cramps without sensory symptoms.

Diffuse weakness without cranial nerve involvement can also suggest a neuromuscular disorder where there has not been prominent

Table 5.1 Clinical approach to weakness and fatigue

Clinical features	Diagnoses
Weakness: one limb	Entrapment neuropathy, radiculopathy. Cerebral lesion less likely
Weakness on one side of the body	Stroke, cerebral mass lesion. Spinal cord lesion less likely
Weakness of the legs	Spinal cord lesion including disk, tumor, demyelinating disease, infarction. Midline parasagittal lesion including mass, bilateral anterior cerebral artery infarctions
Weakness of the entire body including cranial nerves	Neuromuscular disease including ALS, myasthenia gravis. Hypothyroidism
Weakness of the body excluding the cranial nerves	Peripheral neuropathy, hypothyroidism, mid to upper cervical spinal cord lesion
Easy fatigue without weakness	Depression, chronic fatigue syndrome, myasthenia gravis
Tired-all-the-time	Depression, chronic fatigue syndrome

brainstem involvement. Therefore, ALS and myasthenia have to be considered, especially if there are no sensory symptoms. Brisk reflexes and/or Babinski sign suggests ALS, but also can be seen in cervical myelopathy of any cause.

Focal weakness

Focal weakness in one extremity usually suggests an entrapment neuropathy or radiculopathy. Cerebral lesions can cause focal monoparesis, though this is unusual; there are almost always some signs of dysfunction in the other limb on the same side.

Some common and important disorders of focal weakness are as follows:

Arm weakness
- Wrist extension = radial neuropathy.
- Intrinsic muscles of the hand = ulnar neuropathy or C8 radiculopathy.

Leg weakness
- Foot extension/dorsiflexion = peroneal neuropathy or L5 radiculopathy.
- Knee extension = L2–4 radiculopathy or femoral neuropathy.

Hemiparesis
- Dominant side with aphasia = cerebral stroke or mass.
- Dominant side with bulbar signs = brainstem stroke or mass.
- Non-dominant side with neglect, hemianopia = cerebral stroke or mass.
- Non-dominant side with bulbar signs = brainstem stroke or mass.

Paraparesis
- Leg weakness with sensory level and spine pain = spinal cord structural lesion, disk, mass, syrinx.
- Leg weakness with sensory loss, without pain = transverse myelitis, spinal cord infarction, syrinx.
- Leg weakness without pain or sensory loss = transverse myelitis, vitamin B12 deficiency, primary lateral sclerosis

Lack of initiative

Lack of initiative is thought to be the cause for the complaints of weakness and fatigue in several conditions:

- depression
- dementia
- chronic fatigue syndrome.

Add to the lack of initiative a major component of deconditioning and the patient has marked complaints of weakness and fatigue.

Fatigue and tired-all-the-time (TATT)

This is a frequent presenting complaint in family practice.
   The TATT syndrome has three distinct features:

- The declaration of fatigue as the presenting or supporting symptom.
- The miserable, self-pitying tone of voice in which it is expressed: 'I'm just tired, tired all the time' or 'I have got no life in me what-so-ever' or 'I am just thoroughly, thoroughly drained' or 'I'm just like a wet lettuce'.
- The sinking, hopeless feeling in the pit of the stomach of the attending physician.

The important points in the history include:

- time frame: when it started, variation with days of week, time of day, menses;
- presence of other symptoms;
- sleep amount and pattern;
- lifestyle inquiry;
- the patient's own ideas as to its causation;
- the patient's secret fears as to the cause.

It should be quite clear from the questionnaire and a few supplementary questions that the complaint is of fatigue and not of a specific neuromuscular weakness. Note that the questionnaire specifically flag current medications as studies show that at least 5% of TATTs are due to medications. Examination shows no objective weakness, although some components of the motor examination may be effort dependent.

Medical conditions can occasionally cause TATT, although this is rare. Some of the important tests are:

- Serum and urine electrolytes;
- Complete blood count for anemia;
- WBC, ESR, and C-reactive protein (CRP) for infection and inflammatory conditions;
- TSH.

This screen is very cost-effective as it will help dispel any thoughts that the patient has a major physical illness. An in-depth review of the normal results with the patient can greatly alleviate some of the anxiety over the possibility of a serious undiagnosed condition.

How can we help these patients?

This discussion particularly excludes the occasional patients who have a specific medical diagnosis for their fatigue, such as hypothyroidism or renal failure. In the remainder of the patients, they often carry the diagnosis of *chronic fatigue syndrome* (CFS). This is a syndrome rather than a specific diagnosis, and patients fall into three groups. By far the largest are patients with depression and disuse atrophy. The muscular and tissue changes with disuse create some of the symptoms that comprise the accompanying *fibromyalgia syndrome* (FMS). Other patients may have an undiagnosed connective tissue disease or undiagnosed infectious disease.

Some general suggestions for management of these patients:

- Reassure the patient that fatal or disabling conditions have been excluded.
- Advise gentle exercise with an aim to increasing exercise tolerance.
- Consider prescribing an antidepressant. Most patients respond well to SSRIs. Patients with difficulty sleeping at night can be given tricyclic antidepressants as an alternative, although they are poorer antide-

pressants than the SSRIs, causing more side-effects and difficulties with dose-titration. The anxiolytic properties of paroxtine may be useful in promoting sleep.

■ Encourage support groups for patients with similar complaints. This can be extremely helpful, since absence of a sympathetic ear may be an exacerbating factor in these patients.

■ Some patients find it helpful to keep a daily record of their symptoms and observations, since it may psychologically enable them. On the other hand, it might focus the attention of the patient even more on the condition.

Assess patient's lifestyle

Each patient needs to assess the demands on their actions and attentions and prioritize their daily activities.

Sometimes the symptoms are related to the lifestyle the patient leads. He or she is simply unrealistic about their capabilities and expects too much of themselves. This might well be called: 'High Energy Output Failure'.

Human output has its limits and these patients, in states of over-arousal, need to take a step backwards and move back down the graph by altering their over-demanding lifestyles. Their stress is often apparent in their related symptoms – of tension headaches, dizziness, and irritability, which may sound very much like a depression and indeed warrant a trial of SSRIs.

Insight and counseling have a very important role here, and as the prime fault is the over-arousal, adrenergic blocking drugs may also be useful in selected patients.

Counsel the patient on realistic expectations

Counseling is perhaps the only option in patients who are truly 'not as young as they used to be' and haven't yet come to realize it. Again a full examination and screen will be an essential prerequisite to the reassurance that they are physically sound and it may be time to stop and smell the roses and enjoy the bouquets they've earned from their years of toil.

Neurological causes of weakness

Differential diagnosis

Clues to specific locations and diagnoses are made by the neurological exam. The screening exam is sufficient for most complaints, although for evaluation of specific weakness, detailed examination is essential. Anatomical details are essential for this examination. Clinically relevant anatomical details are presented in the Appendix.

Cerebral causes are suggested by disorders of consciousness or cortical functions, including language, vision, memory, or personality.

Spinal cord location is suggested by weakness of the legs or legs and arms without any bulbar or cerebral signs. Pain is common with most causes of myelopathy, although not all. Likewise, a sensory level on the trunk is common but not invariable.

A *plexus* lesion is suggested by weakness in one limb, which spans individual nerve or root distributions. Most lesions of the plexus are painful.

Peripheral nerve or root lesion is suggested by weakness in the distribution of a single peripheral nerve or nerve root. Sensory symptoms or signs or reflex abnormality can be supportive, but again is not invariable.

Weakness and fatigability with normal or depressed reflexes suggest neuromuscular causes of weakness. Distal weakness suggests neuronal or axonal damage. Proximal weakness suggests muscle or neuromuscular junction dysfunction.

Cerebral causes
Vascular disease
Stroke produces weakness of sudden onset. Some strokes have a progressive or stuttering onset, though this is unusual. More

commonly, the weakness develops suddenly or is noted upon arising. Chapter 9 presents details on diagnosis and treatment of stroke.

Weakness due to stroke has a distribution, which depends on the vessel involved:

Anterior cerebral arteries (ACA)

ACA infarction produces weakness, which is most prominent in the contralateral leg. The right and left ACAs may have a common origin, so bilateral infarction is possible producing bilateral leg weakness which can be mistaken for myelopathy.

Middle cerebral artery (MCA)

MCA infarction produces weakness, which is most prominent in the contralateral arm, although the leg is commonly affected to a lesser extent. Other signs of cortical dysfunction are also seen, including aphasia for dominant hemisphere lesions and neglect with non-dominant hemisphere lesions.

Posterior cerebral arteries (PCA)

PCA infarction produces mainly visual loss with a contralateral hemianopia. Memory deficit is also common as branches of the PCA supply the mesial temporal lobe.

Vertebro-basilar arteries

Vertebral occlusion may produce the lateral medullary (Wallenberg's) syndrome, which is usually caused by occlusion of the posterior inferior cerebellar artery. Basilar thrombosis produces quadriparesis with brainstem dysfunction.

Lenticulostriate arteries

The lenticulostriate arteries are branches of the proximal portion of the MCA. These are small penetrating vessels which supply the basal ganglia and internal capsule. Infarction in the distribution of these vessels produces contralateral hemiparesis, which affects the arm, face and leg, about equally. Cortical symptoms are distinctly absent.

Thalamoperforate arteries

The thalamoperforate arteries are branches of the PCA and supply the thalamus. These are also penetrating vessels which can be responsible for lacunar infarction. Contralateral sensory loss and/or thalamic pain syndrome can result. Weakness can be present as well, although this is less prominent than with lenticulostriate infarction.

Mass lesion

Mass lesions can occur anywhere in the cerebral hemispheres. Unfortunately, localization on the basis of clinical presentation alone is quite imperfect but there is some localizing value to clinical symptoms and signs.

Frontal lobe

Frontal lobe lesions typically produce apathy with lack of initiative rather than paralysis. Posterior frontal lesions may involve the motor strip and association areas, thereby producing weakness. The region of weakness depends on the part of the motor strip involved, with midline/parasagittal lesions producing leg weakness and laterally placed hemispheric lesions producing arm and face weakness, usually with signs of cortical dysfunction, as discussed above.

Temporal lobe

Temporal lobe lesions seldom produce weakness of any kind. Dominant hemisphere temporal lobe lesions can produce fluent aphasias. Non-dominant temporal lobe lesions may be clinically silent.

Parietal lobe

Parietal lobe lesions produce sensory deficits more than motor deficits. Anterior parietal lesions can affect the posterior aspect of the motor strip, producing weakness, which depends on the location of the lesion. Parasagittal lesions produce leg weakness and lateral lesions produce arm weakness.

Occipital lobe

Occipital lobe lesions usually do not cause weakness, although distal branches of the posterior cerebral arteries supply deep nuclei, infarction of which can produce motor deficit.

Posterior fossa

Mass lesions in the posterior fossa produce the combination of limb weakness and bulbar signs. The weakness is usually a quadriparesis rather than a hemiparesis. Bulbar signs include dysarthria and/or dysphagia, diplopia, and facial weakness.

Speed of growth

Slowly growing lesions tend to produce irritation of surrounding neurons so that seizures are common. Quickly growing lesions are less likely to produce seizures because they are typically destructive. More common symptoms are focal deficits. Headache and confusion can occur from increased intracranial pressure associated with a rapidly growing lesion. Slowly growing lesions are much less likely to produce increased intracranial pressure unless there is obstruction of ventricular outflow.

Multiple sclerosis (MS)

Patients with MS have a tendency to have diffuse fatigue in addition to any objective neurological weakness. However, diffuse fatigue without other neurological complaints is not an expected presenting complaint leading to the diagnosis of MS. If the neurological examination shows no objective abnormalities, then evaluation for MS is not warranted.

Common symptoms which lead to the diagnosis of MS include:

- diplopia
- ataxia
- paraparesis
- visual loss
- hemiparesis.

Virtually all patients being evaluated for MS need neurological consultation. After diagnosis has been established and treatment initiated, the general physician often follows these patients, monitoring therapy, if given, and treating medical complications such as urinary tract infection (UTI) and upper respiratory infection (URI). The generalist may also feel comfortable treating acute attacks and managing spasticity of the patients after this initial phase of treatment.

Diagnosis

The key to diagnosis is the identification of deficits that cannot be explained by a single lesion in the nervous system. This identification of multiple lesions narrows the differential diagnosis to a few entities:

- MS
- vasculitis and other causes of multifocal infarctions
- lupus
- multiple metastases.

A second key to diagnosis is having episodic symptoms. Most patients who are diagnosed with MS will have had previous episodes of neurological deficit as listed above. However, the episodes may not have received medical attention or might nor have been recognized as being due to demyelinating disease. Therefore, careful questioning of patients with suspected MS is essential.

MRI is more sensitive then CT for the diagnosis of MS, as demyelinating plaques will usually not be visualized on CT. Either imaging technique can rule-out multiple mass lesions and infarctions.

Treatment

There are three ways to treat MS:

- treat the acute attack;
- reduce the frequency of attacks;
- treat the symptoms.

Treatment of acute attacks usually consists of administration of steroids. These agents have been proven to shorten an attack when given intravenously. Oral steroids are not used except as a follow-up treatment to intravenous treatment for optic neuritis. Most experts recommend administration of methylprednisolone 1 g i.v. daily for 5 days. If the deficit is optic neuritis, this is followed by a tapering dose of oral steroids, usually as prednisolone. Treatment of the acute attack shortens the attack but does not improve the level of recovery which can be expected. In addition, it does not alter the frequency of subsequent attacks. There has been some concern that the frequency of attacks may actually be increased by administration of steroids, but with treatment as outlined here, this is not expected.

Reducing the frequency of attacks is best accomplished by one of the interferons, glatiramer acetate or mitaxanthrone. Unfortunately, these agents are not available to all patients, although, arguably, they should be.

Treating the symptoms in MS consists of addressing these fundamental symptoms:

- diplopia
- spasticity
- ataxia
- fatigue.

Diplopia is treated by patching one eye. It is recommended to not consistently patch the same eye, but rather alternating on successive days. After the initial phase of recovery, persistent diplopia can be treated by special prism glasses, although these should not be purchased too soon, since many patients improve well.

Spasticity is treated by any of several medicines discussed in the section on spasticity presented in Chapter 11. Baclofen is the most commonly used drug, with diazepam being a close second. Patients usually adapt to the cognitive slowing which develops after initiation of these drugs.

Ataxia has no good treatment, although amantadine is frequently tried. This produces improvement for a minority of patients, but some do feel it helps. Since it is also used for fatigue of MS, this treatment is worthwhile to try.

Among patients with MS who do complain of fatigue, there are a few self-help guidelines which we recommend. In addition, two medicines have been used with some degree of efficacy:

- Amantadine
- Modafanil.

Each of these agents can be tried when the diagnosis is certain, but should not be used as a therapeutic trial when there is not a defined neurological diagnosis.

Spinal cord diseases

Common disorders of the spinal cord can produce weakness. Associated findings can suggest the diagnosis, although structural imaging is required for most patients with myelopathy.

Transverse myelitis

Transverse myelitis is one of a number of restricted inflammatory disorders that affect the nervous system. Transverse myelitis presents with the subacute onset of paraparesis and often leg pain. There may not be any back pain, which would argue against a structural lesion of the spine. Some patients with transverse myelitis go on to develop other signs of demyelination, including optic neuritis or demyelination elsewhere in the brain.

All patients with acute onset of paraplegia or quadriplegia without signs of cranial nerve deficit require MRI or myelogram to look for compressive lesion of the spinal cord. A good-quality contrast-enhanced MRI can usually show the area of cord inflammation in patients with transverse myelitis, although this is not invariable.

Patients with transverse myelitis are usually treated with intravenous corticosteroids, as are patients with an attack of MS. However, the scientific evidence to support this is not strong. This should be the province of the consultant neurologist for making the diagnosis and initiating therapy.

Neoplastic spinal cord compression

Neoplastic spinal cord compression produces weakness of the legs, usually with severe back pain. In retrospect, the back pain predates the weakness. Clinical findings depend on the level of the lesion, with lesions of the thoracic and cervical spine producing pyramidal tract signs in the legs, and those of the lumbar spine producing leg weakness with bowel/bladder dysfunction and areflexia, suggesting a conus medullaris or cauda equina lesion. Cervical spine lesions typically produce arm weakness in addition to the leg weakness.

Infarction of the spinal cord

Infarction of the spinal cord is most common in the thoracic area, with occlusion of the anterior spinal artery. The anterior two-thirds of the cord are damaged with prominent loss of motor function below the level of the lesion plus loss of pain and temperature sensation. Vibration and proprioception are relatively preserved, since the anterior spinal artery does not supply the dorsal columns.

Subacute combined degeneration

Subacute combined degeneration from vitamin B12 deficiency results in clinical findings of peripheral neuropathy and/or myelopathy; differing findings may predominate in different patients.

Macrocytic anemia and peripheral neuropathy are not invariable findings in patients with B12 deficiency. Therefore, this diagnosis should be considered even in patients without signs of these associated conditions.

Vitamin B12 replacement results in improvement in ataxia and strength, but the improvement is often not complete. This emphasizes the importance of early diagnosis to make for an optimal outcome.

Spondylitic myelopathy

Spondylitic damage to the spinal column is most prominent in the lumbar and cervical levels. When the cervical spine is involved, weakness in the legs is associated with corticospinal tract signs, and weakness in the arms is associated with reflex loss at the level of the lesion. When the damage is in the lumbar spine, weakness in the legs is accompanied by loss of reflexes.

Syrinx

Syringomyelia produces weakness of the legs with corticospinal tract signs. Arm symptoms often precede the leg symptoms and include loss of pain and temperature sensation across the shoulders and upper arms.

Diagnosis is made by MRI or myelography. Treatment depends on the type of syrinx. If the syrinx is due to compression of the rostral spinal cord by a Chiari malformation, then surgical decompression of the Chiari malformation will improve the syrinx. Otherwise, direct decompression of the syrinx may be performed. As with other causes of compressive myelopathy, early treatment is the key as reversal of the pressure effect allows the neurons to repair themselves, but recovery is often incomplete.

Neuromuscular diseases

Neuromuscular diseases are differentiated from most spinal cord disorders by absence of hyperactive reflexes. In fact, reflexes may be decreased in most diseases except for ALS.

Neuropathy

Peripheral neuropathy produces distal weakness with atrophy, which is first obvious in the intrinsic muscles of the feet and then hands. The tibialis anterior is often affected. Sensory symptoms include dysesthesias, paresthesias, burning pain, and sensory loss. The sensory loss may not be obvious, but sharp-dull differentiation and vibration are often affected.

Diagnosis is by clinical presentation. EMG can be confirmatory but does not always identify small fiber and sensory neuropathies.

Radiculopathy

Radiculopathy is more likely to produce sensory loss than weakness, and when weakness is present, it is much less prominent than the sensory findings and pain. Therefore, radiculopathy is discussed in detail in Chapter 6. In brief:

- Weakness of the biceps suggests C6 radiculopathy.
- Weakness of the wrist and finger extensors suggests C7 radiculopathy or radial neuropathy.
- Weakness of the triceps suggests C7 radiculopathy, although proximal radial neuropathy can produce this, as well.
- Weakness of extension of the great toe is the most sensitive finding suggesting L5 radiculopathy.

Weakness with S1 radiculopathy is usually not prominent because the gastrocnemii are so strong. The most sensitive sign is loss of the Achilles reflex, although this is not specific, since neuropathy can produce the same finding, and the Achilles reflex is commonly depressed or absent in elderly patients.

Motorneuron disease

Motorneuron diseases include ALS and a small number of related conditions. Patients present with weakness without any sensory findings. The most important motorneuron diseases are:

- Amyotrophic lateral sclerosis
- Primary lateral sclerosis
- Spinal muscular atrophy

The key to differentiating ALS from other neuromuscular causes of weakness is increased tendon reflexes and upgoing plantar response (Babinski sign).

Primary lateral sclerosis produces weakness of the legs without involvement of the arms and without sensory abnormalities to suggest transverse myelitis.

Spinal muscular atrophy is a degeneration of the lower motorneuron which typically appears in infancy or childhood, therefore is not really in the differential diagnosis of ALS. Reflexes are not increased.

Myasthenia gravis

Myasthenia presents with weakness, which is most prominent later in the day and relatively improved in the morning and after a rest. Ptosis and diplopia associated with otherwise normal brainstem function is typical, and strongly supports the diagnosis. Differentiation of individual cranial neuropathies from neuromuscular weakness, which spans neural distribution, is crucial to the diagnosis. Examination is best if each eye is first tested individually.

The following tests are commonly performed in patients with suspected myasthenia gravis:

- acetylcholine receptor binding antibody;
- EMG with repetitive stimulation;
- edrophonium test.

The general physician usually does not perform these tests. The edrophonium test consists of administering a small dose of this cholinesterase inhibitor intravenously, while observing the patient for improvement in weakness, usually of eye movements and ptosis. Improvement usually develops in a few minutes. Acute worsening or cardiovascular complications are uncommon but can occur, so this should not be performed in the clinic without resuscitative equipment.

If myasthenia gravis is diagnosed a CT of the chest is performed to look for thymoma. If thymoma is present, it is surgically removed. In some patients the thymus is removed even if no thymoma is found; however, this approach is controversial.

Treatment options for myasthenia gravis include:

- prednisolone
- pyridostigmine
- azathioprine
- IVIg
- plasmapheresis.

Other immune suppressants can be used, although these are the most commonly employed. Definitive diagnosis and treatment of myasthenia gravis is begun by the neurologist. The generalist will follow the patient after the phase of acute treatment and will usually inherit a patient who is on tapering doses of prednisolone along with some sort of GI protection and pyridostigmine. Dosing of the prednisolone will probably be formulated by the specialist, but in general, alternate day dosing will be the goal; reducing to the minimum amount needed to stabilize the patient.

Pyridostigmine is a short-acting cholinesterase inhibitor which is used to improve strength of the patients while the immune-modulating therapy eventually controls the disease. Increasing doses of pyridostigmine improves strength up to a maximum effect. Higher doses can make the patient weaker again. Therefore, patients and generalists need to be aware of this effect so the weakness produced by excessive doses does not trigger self-administration of even higher doses.

Polymyositis

Polymyositis is one of a family of inflammatory myopathies, which presents with proximal weakness without sensory deficit. Some patients have pain, but this is not universal, despite the '...itis' of the name. Diagnosis is considered in any patients of any age with proximal weakness.

Laboratory findings in polymyositis include:

- elevated creatine kinase;
- EMG signs of myopathy;
- muscle biopsy signs of inflammation and muscle fiber degeneration.

Not all of these features need to be present for the diagnosis, but two of the three are required for initiation of treatment.

Treatment for polymyositis is usually with prednisolone, although other immune modulators are also occasionally used. Confirmation of the diagnosis and initiation of treatment is typically by a neurologist or rheumatologist. Subsequently, the patient returns to the general physician on tapering doses of prednisolone with GI protection. The goal is to eventually taper the patient onto a low alternating day dose of steroids.

Weakness may become worse during treatment for polymyositis. The important question at this point is: Is the weakness an exacerbation of polymyositis or due to steroid myopathy? The answer to this question is crucial since treatment would be totally different. If the polymyositis has become active again, then increasing the steroid dose is required. If the weakness is due to steroid myopathy, then more rapid tapering of the steroids should be attempted. Again, the consultant can help with this assessment and might perform a follow-up EMG to help with differentiation; however, creatine kinase (CK) determination may be helpful. Markedly elevated CK argues in favor of reactivation of disease whereas normal CK argues in favor of steroid myopathy.

Botulism

Botulism presents with autonomic symptoms including abdominal cramps, diarrhea, and constipation. This is followed by generalized weakness with ocular and bulbar involvement. The initial GI distress is the key to suspicion.

Confirmation of diagnosis and initiation of treatment for botulism is completely in the realm of the neurologist. All patients with suspected botulism should be referred for emergent care. This is never a disease that can be followed from a distance.

Eaton–Lambert syndrome

Eaton–Lambert myasthenic syndrome is a rare paraneoplastic disorder, that produces proximal or generalized weakness. Key to suspicion is autonomic symptoms including dry mouth and impotence, although these findings are less prominent than with botulism.

Confirmation of the diagnosis of Eaton–Lambert syndrome is by measurement of the titer of antibodies to a particular voltage-gated calcium channel. This is often included as part of a *paraneoplastic panel* which tests for this and other paraneoplastic antibodies. Diagnosis of Eaton–Lambert syndrome requires vigorous search for underlying malignancy, especially small cell lung cancer. The neuromuscular disease may predate identification of the cancer by up to two years, so if the initial evaluation is negative, the patient must be restudied at intervals of about three months for the two years. Chest CT is typically done at these times. Chest x-ray is not adequate for visualizing especially small tumors.

Non-neurological causes

Depression

Depression is a common ultimate diagnosis in patients with complaints of weakness, fatigue, and even memory loss. Typical signs of depression are present including:

- change in sleep pattern (more or less);
- change in food intake (more or less);
- crying, depressed mood;
- lack of full participation in family and occupational activities.

Although formal criteria for the diagnosis of depression exist, in the context of generalized tiredness, the suspicion of a depressive illness warrants a therapeutic trial of the most appropriate SSRI. Careful explanation and follow-up will ensure that patient outcome is best served by this approach.

Depression may accompany many medical and neurological disorders, so the diagnosis of depression should not lull the physician into complacency, to be caught napping while a serious illness is undiagnosed.

Chronic fatigue syndrome

Chronic fatigue syndrome is not a disease, but a combination of symptoms including muscle weakness and pain, headache, sensory symptoms including pain and paresthesias. Other symptoms including memory loss, dizziness, and even fainting are common. Diagnosis is established merely by the symptoms of muscle fatigue for at least 6 months.

There are reports of biochemical abnormalities in patients with chronic fatigue syndrome and the related syndrome – fibromyalgia. However, many clinicians still do not ascribe disease status to these vague entities. Many feel that chronic fatigue syndrome is related to lack of initiative and deconditioning, often with depression as a prime component.

These patients may respond well to antidepressants that are often started at half the usual dosage. Adequate sleep is probably also important.

Medical conditions
Thyroid disorders

Hypothyroidism is also associated with complaints of diffuse fatigue, and patients may seem depressed. However, associated findings including abnormalities of hair and skin. Tendon reflexes are slow to elicit and slow to relax.

Hyperthyroidism is also associated with complaints of weakness, although the stigmata of hyperthyroidism are often more readily identified than those of hypothyroidism. Nevertheless, some patients with thyroid storm may present with weakness and encephalopathy without other stigmata of hyperthyroidism.

Adrenal disorders

Cushing's syndrome often presents with weakness, regardless of whether it is drug-induced or due to adrenal disorder. With chronic hypercortisolism, central obesity with limb wasting is common.

Falls in the elderly

Falls in the elderly are usually multifactorial with some of the important contributing factors being:

- impaired postural reflexes
- visual loss
- loss of vestibular function
- decreased proprioceptive sensation
- extremity weakness.

All of these are normal accompaniment to aging, but can be exacerbated in a many disease states including:

- peripheral neuropathy
- Parkinsonism
- cerebrovascular disease
- macular degeneration or cataracts
- dementia
- alcoholism
- cardiac arrhythmia
- congestive heart failure (CHF).

Important points to ask on history are:

- Is there loss of consciousness?
- Do you fall over even while sitting?

■ Can you walk better in the bright light vs. darkened room?

Important findings to look for on examination include:

■ normal and tandem gait;
■ Romberg testing;
■ visual fields and acuity;
■ position sense in the legs;
■ mental status;
■ muscle tone and limb movement;
■ cardiac auscultation;
■ orthostatic blood pressures.

Laboratory study of patients with frequent unexplained falls should include:

■ CT head
■ ECG
■ vitamin B12 level
■ thyroid function tests.

A single cause for falls in the elderly is not frequently found, and there is no treatment if a reversible cause is not identified. There are a number of suggestions to be given to patients, however, which may improve their ambulation:

■ walk next to a wall when possible;
■ use a cane or quad-cane;

Pearls
■ Generalized fatigue with a normal blood screen is rarely due to an identifiable pathology.
■ Depression is the single most frequent diagnosis.
■ A second opinion may be needed to head off an 'impasse' when the patient won't accept the diagnosis.
■ Focal weakness may be embellished, especially if the real deficit is mild. Take care to not immediately dismiss the complaint as psychosomatic.

- have lights on when walking, perhaps requiring night lights in the house;
- stand beside the bed or chair for a minute or two before walking;
- if symptoms of presyncope develop, sit down immediately, even if on the floor.

When to refer

- When the clinical findings suggest myopathy or neuromuscular transmission abnormality, referral to neurology is warranted because confirmatory tests need to be done.
- When focal weakness suggests a new or evolving structural lesion – neurology or neurosurgery.
- Generalized weakness with no sensory symptoms or signs suggests myopathy, neuromuscular transmission defect, or motorneuron disease. These findings with brisk reflexes suggest motorneuron disease such as ALS.

chapter 6

Sensory disorders

Overview

Sensory deficits can involve:

- Somatosensory information
- Visual information
- Auditory information.

Somatosensory details are discussed first, followed by discussion of visual and auditory deficits.

Physiology of sensory systems

Sensation is transduced into neuronal signals by a variety of receptors, from specialized organs to bare nerve endings. The final common pathway to activation of these nerves is deformation of the nerve endings which results in depolarization of the nerve terminal. The depolarization creates a generator potential which then results in action potentials in the afferent sensory nerve.

Somatosensory neurons ascend to the spinal cord and separate into two main divisions. Pain and temperature sensation ascend mostly crossed in the spinothalamic tract. The neurons making up these axons are association neurons in the spinal cord segments. Vibration and proprioception ascends in the posterior columns. These neurons are the central projections of the dorsal root ganglia neurons, with their peripheral processes extending to the periphery of the body.

Table 6.1 Definition of somatosensory terms

Term	Definition	Cause?
Allodynia	Misperception such that non-noxious stimuli are perceived as painful	Sensory processing usually at the thalamic level misinterprets sensory input as painful when it should be non-painful
Anesthesia	Absence of sensory perception	Absence of relay of sensory information to consciousness. Origin may be at any level, from peripheral nerve, spine, brain sensory pathways, or medication-induced unconsciousness of the patient
Dysesthesia	Abnormal perception of a sensory stimulus, such as when pressure or light touch induces tingling	Stimulation of a nerve results in multiple action potentials when one or a few would have normally been elicited. The depolarization is prolonged
Hyperesthesia	Exaggerated sensory perception, as when a light touch evokes a strong cutaneous sensation	Damaged sensory neurons at any level produce a volley of action potentials in response to stimulation which would normally evoke fewer discharges
Hypoesthesia	Decreased sensory perception	Decreased numbers of functioning sensory neurons and impaired generation of action potentials produces decreased perception of sensory stimuli

Table 6.1 continued

Term	Definition	Cause?
Paresthesia	Abnormal spontaneous sensation, usually tingling or itching	Fluctuating membrane potentials of damaged nerves result in episodic action potentials which can occur in bursts
Analgesia	Absence of perception of noxious stimuli	Small fiber neuropathy (e.g. amylordosis; syrinx)
Hypalgesia	Decreased perception of noxious stimuli	Small fiber neuropathy (e.g. amyloid; diabetes)
Hyperalgesia (hyperpathia)	Exaggerated sensory perception of noxious stimuli	Large fiber neuropathy causing imbalance of noxious and non-noxious sensory information reaching the spinal cord and/or brain stem from the periphery

The dorsal column axons ascend to the cervico-medullary junction where they synapse in the nucleus cuneatus (for the arm) and nucleus gracilis (for the leg). The second order neurons cross and ascend through the brainstem and synapse in the thalamus. Neurons from the spinothalamic tract and dorsal column project to different regions of the thalamus.

Visual information travels in the optic nerves to the optic chiasm where about half of the fibers cross. The optic tracts carry visual information from the contralateral hemifield to the occipital lobe via a thalamic relay.

Auditory information travels through the acoustic nerve (VIII) to the brainstem where it ascends bilaterally to the midbrain. Then, the information is relayed to the temporal lobes via a thalamic relay for cortical interpretation.

Terminology

The terminology of somatosensory sensory loss is a bit confusing but needs to be clarified so that we can all understand the terms used in discussion of sensory deficit. Table 6.1 shows some common terms for sensory loss.

Approach to the patient

Diagnosis of sensory disturbance depends on accurate localization of the lesion. Localization of the lesion depends on description of the sensory deficit and examination for non-sensory deficit.

Table 6.2 shows some of the common causes of sensory disorders and their differentiating features.

Somatosensory complaints

Peripheral causes

Sensory polyneuropathy

Sensory neuropathy is common and frequently undiagnosed. Patients rarely come to the doctor with numbness in the absence of pain, they are more likely to seek medical attention for pain as a sensory symptom or weakness as a motor symptom.

Sensory neuropathy may be due to many causes but some important ones are:

- HIV neuropathy
- hereditary neuropathy
- some toxins
- amyloid
- diabetes mellitus.

Diabetes produces a neuropathy which can initially have mainly sensory features, but motor deficits eventually develop with wasting of intrinsic muscles of the hands and feet.

Table 6.2 Sensory disorders

Disorder	Features	Causes
Loss of taste (ageusia)	Loss of elementary taste sensation	Bell's palsy, less likely a brainstem lesion
Loss of smell (anosmia)	Loss of pure smell sensation	Trauma, olfactory groove meningioma, Parkinsonism
Cutaneous sensory loss on one limb	Alteration in sensation on one limb, usually involving just part of a limb	Peripheral nerve, plexus, or root lesion. Exact distribution is key to diagnosis
Cutaneous sensory loss on one side of the body	Loss or alteration of sensation on face, arm, and leg of one side	Thalamic or hemispheric lesion
Cutaneous sensation loss on both legs	Sensory level seen as sharp sensation is tested proceeding down the body	Spinal cord lesion, regardless of cause

Amyloid produces a neuropathy that is most prominently sensory. While motor symptoms can develop, they are typically eclipsed by the sensory findings.

Most sensory neuropathies present with sensory deficit, but the symptom which usually triggers a visit to the physician is often pain. Most patients have a phase of their condition when pain is prominent, although subsequently the pain usually abates, as the small sensory fibers that carries noxious stimuli are completely destroyed.

Carpal tunnel syndrome

Carpal tunnel syndrome is the most common mononeuropathy. The cause is compression of the median nerve at the wrist, under the transverse carpal ligament. Certain medical disorders predispose to carpal tunnel syndrome, including obesity, rheumatoid arthritis, acromegaly, hypothyroidism, and other causes of peripheral neuropathy.

Patients present with numbness of the palm which involving digits 1–3 without involvement of 4–5. Pain in the wrist and hand is common, although the non-noxious sensory abnormalities may predate the pain by months to years. Sensory symptoms are exacerbated during sustained hand grip such as driving and during sleep; patients often awake with palm pain and numbness.

Ulnar neuropathy

The two most common causes of ulnar neuropathy are compression near the elbow and diabetes. This is the most common mononeuropathy seen with diabetes.

Patients present with numbness, dysesthesias, and often pain in digits 4–5. The ulnar-side of digit 4 is mainly involved. Pain may extend into the forearm but sensory deficit should not, since the ulnar nerve distal to the elbow does not supply cutaneous sensation to the forearm.

Meralgia paresthetica

Meralgia paresthetica is due to damage to the lateral femoral cutaneous nerve. The most common area of damage is where the nerve passes beneath the inguinal ligament as it passes from the

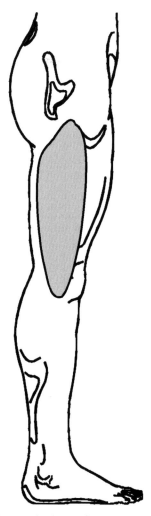

Figure 6.1 *Sensory distribution for meralgia paresthetica.*

pelvis to the thigh. Pregnancy, obesity, and certain occupational activities predispose to damage to this nerve (Fig. 6.1).

Patients present with pain and numbness on the lateral aspect of the thigh. The distribution of the symptoms is critical. If the sensory symptoms extend below the knee or wrap onto the medial aspect of the leg, then the diagnosis is not meralgia paresthetica.

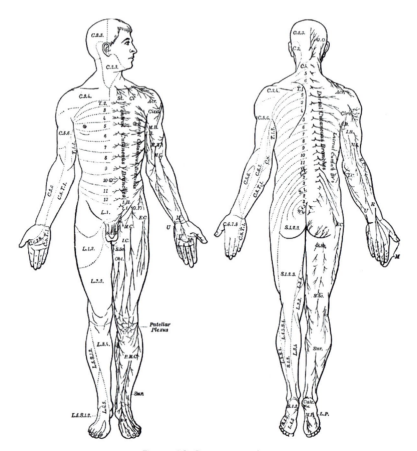

Figure 6.2 *Dermatome chart.*

Spinal causes

Radiculopathy

Radiculopathy at any level can produce sensory disturbance, and the distribution may not conform exactly to the dermatomal diagrams (Fig. 6.2). The sensory disturbance may be dysesthesias and paresthesias, hypoesthesia, and/or shooting or stabbing pain.

The most common radiculopathies are due to intervertebral disc disease, and therefore the most common radicular sensory symptoms are C6, C7, L5, and S1. Diabetic radiculopathy can be at any level,

Table 6.3 Radiculopathies

Level	Motor findings	Sensory findings	Reflex change
Cervical radiculopathy			
C5	Deltoid, biceps	Radial forearm	Biceps
C6	Biceps, brachioradialis	Digits 1 and 2	Biceps
C7	Wrist extensors, triceps	Digits 3 and 4	Triceps
C8	Intrinsic hand muscles	Digit 5	Commonly none
Lumbar radiculopathy			
L2	Psoas, quadriceps	Lateral and anterior upper thigh	Knee
L3	Psoas, quadriceps	Lower medial thigh	Knee
L4	Tibialis anterior, quadriceps	Medial lower leg	Knee
L5	Peroneus longus, gluteus medius, tibialis anterior, toe extension	Lateral lower leg	None
S1	Gastrocnemius, gluteus maximus	Lateral foot, digits 4 and 5, outside of sole	Achilles/ankle

with 50% occurring in thoracic dermatomes. Thoracic radiculopathy from primary spinal disease is uncommon.

Table 6.3 presents the common motor and sensory findings in patients with radiculopathy. Most of the symptoms are sensory, so this condition is discussed here, although weakness can also develop and when present suggests surgical consultation is indicated.

The most common cervical radiculopathy involves C7. This presents with numbness of digits 3 and 4 of the hand and is associated with weakness of the triceps and sometimes of the wrist (the triceps weakness can be so prominent that in several patients who were darts players the unexpected loss of power meant that the dart failed to reach the dartboard, to their great embarrassment). This can be confused with radial neuropathy, but with the latter the weakness is much more prominent. Weakness of the wrist to the point of wrist drop is much more likely related to radial neuropathy than C7 radiculopathy.

The most common lumbosacral radiculopathy is L5–S1 with entrapment of the S1 nerve root. Patients present with sensory loss on the outside of the foot and loss of the Achilles reflex. L5 radiculopathy is next in frequency, and these patients present with sensory loss on the lateral aspect of the lower leg without a reflex abnormality. Extension of the great toe is the most sensitive sign of L5 radiculopathy.

Syrinx

A syrinx is a fluid-filled cyst in the spinal cord that extends over several segments. The most common causes are the Chiari II (Arnold Chiari) malformation or the Chiari I malformation in which the cerebellar tonsils extend downward into the top of the cervical spine. This causes obstruction of flow within the central canal with subsequent dilation. The pressure effect initially affects the crossing fibers of the spinothalamic tract but can subsequently affect other ascending and descending axons.

Patients present with loss of pain and temperature sensation at the levels of the lesion. With the most common location in the cervical spine, the sensory loss is in a cape-like distribution across the shoulders. Spasticity can develop below the level of the lesion, and this is the symptom which usually draws the patient to evaluation.

Central causes

Stroke

The most common cause of sensory disturbance with stroke is infarction or hemorrhage of the thalamus. The thalamus is supplied by the thalamoperforate arteries, which are branches of the posterior cerebral arteries. These vessels separate from the main trunk of the posterior cerebral artery proximal to the supply to the occipital lobes.

Thalamic infarct is almost always a lacunar event – due to occlusion of one of the penetrating branches. Symptoms usually are prominently sensory, although some motor and even language function can be affected.

Thalamic pain syndrome (Dejerine-Roussy)

Thalamic pain could be considered in the chapter on pain (Chapter 7) but sensory deficit typically precedes the development of pain and is a prominent clue to diagnosis. The cause is typically infarction involving the thalamoperforate branches of the posterior cerebral artery.

Patients present with sensory deficit on one side of the body. The loss will span extremities, indicating that the lesion is not at the spinal or cortical level. After the initial sensory deficit, pain and hypersensitivity to even light touch (allodynia) develops.

Treatment of thalamic pain is usually tried with anticonvulsants. Carbamazepine and gabapentin are mainly used, although others can be used as well. Tricyclic antidepressant drugs (e.g. amitriptyline) may also be helpful.

Multiple sclerosis

Multiple sclerosis can present with a variety of neurological findings, but among the most common are sensory loss on the face and extremities. Occasionally, patients may present with facial numbness which may be misdiagnosed as trigeminal neuralgia; however, in trigeminal neuralgia, sensory loss is distinctly absent.

Numbness of the extremities is often a sign of myelopathy associated with MS, and may occur in the absence of frank motor and reflex signs of myelopathy. Patients with reports of numbness and no objective signs on neurological examination seldom have a serious condition. However, MS should be considered, especially if the sensory disturbance can easily be explained by a focal neurological lesion.

Medical causes of numbness and tingling

Renal failure

Renal failure results in a sensorimotor neuropathy with prominent early sensory involvement. Patients present with dysesthesias and muscle cramps. Restless legs is a common presenting complaint. Sensory findings are prominent early in the disorder and motor deficit is often not present.

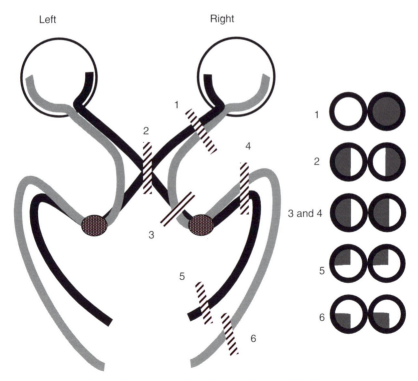

Figure 6.3 *Anatomical localization of visual field defects.*

Drug reactions

Some drugs can cause peripheral neuropathy and thereby produce a sensory deficit. Chemotherapeutic drugs are the most common culprits, and the neuropathy can be dose-limiting. The list of drugs which can potentially produce neuropathy is exhaustive, but the most important are cisplatin and vincristine. The neuropathy of cisplatin can worsen even weeks after cessation of the drug. However, eventually, most chemotherapy-induced neuropathies improve although not to normal.

Visual complaints

Visual defects can usually be accurately localized by examination. The most common visual complaints are:

- blurred vision
- loss of vision in one eye
- loss of vision to one side (hemianopia).

Figure 6.3 shows the anatomic defects which would produce some common visual field abnormalities. Table 6.4 summarizes the responsible lesions and causes.

Blurred vision

The most important causes of blurred vision are:

- refractive error
- glaucoma
- retinal detachment.

These are ophthalmological causes that should be addressed by an ophthalmologist. Unfortunately, patients with retinal detachment may not have a defined visual field abnormality and the area of detachment may not be visible on the general physician's eye exam. Neurological causes can also produce blurred vision, but less so than monocular visual loss.

Table 6.4 Visual field defects

Field defect	Location	Common causes
Right hemianopia	Left optic tract, optic radiation, or occipital lobe	Compressive lesion, left MCA stroke, left PCA stroke
Macular-sparing right hemianopia	Occipital lobe, pole supplied by MCA is spared	Left PCA stroke, macular region supplied by MCA
Hemianopia	Loss of vision to one side, using both eyes	Unilateral optic tract or occipital lesion
Superior quadrant defect	Loss of vision in the upper visual field on one side of both eyes	Lesion of the temporal lobe or lower bank of the visual cortex
Inferior quadrant defect	Loss of vision in the lower visual field on one side of both eyes	Lesion of the parietal lobe or upper bank of the visual cortex
Monocular visual loss	Loss of vision in the entire visual field of only one eye	Lesion of the eye or optic nerve. If transient, suggests vascular insufficiency
Bitemporal hemianopia	Loss of vision in the temporal fields of both eyes, when tested independently	Pituitary tumor, chiasmal lesion
Binasal hemianopia	Loss of vision in the nasal fields of both eyes when tested independently	Lesion around the sella, especially tumor

Monocular visual loss

The most common neurological causes of monocular visual loss are ischemia and optic neuritis. Optic nerve and chiasma compression can also produce visual loss, but this is rare in general practice, and almost always associated with severe pain.

Ischemia is the most common cause of monocular visual loss that is seen by neurologists. Microemboli are thought to come mainly from the carotid artery. Transient monocular blindness (TMB) or amaurosis fugax is essentially a TIA where the ischemia involves the eye and not the rest of the brain. Patients may see a shade descend or ascend across the visual field. Duration of the visual loss is usually minutes. Patients with TMB need evaluation for TIA as described in Chapter 9.

Optic neuritis is characterized by the development of visual loss over hours to days. This differs from ischemia where the onset is sudden.

Hemianopia

In practice, few patients complain of a hemianopia but this is often identified on examination. Patients are often surprised when they are found to be unable to see to one side. In fact, they may claim that the visual loss is not present despite proof.

Hemianopia is easiest to identify with double simultaneous stimulation. The patient looks at the face of the examiner as the examiner holds hands up on each side; the upper and lower quadrants are tested. The patient is asked to count the fingers on both hands. The presentation of double simultaneous stimuli is more sensitive then testing each quadrant in turn. Inability to see an object when there is a competing visual stimulus in the opposite visual field suggest a parietal, rather than occipital, process.

Auditory complaints

Vibrations in the air induce vibration in the tympanic membrane. This vibration is then transmitted mechanically by the ossicles then cochlea through the oval window. Vibration of the oval window produces movement of the perilymph and basilar membrane. Hair cells are stimulated by movement of the membrane. The membrane is sonotopically organized with high frequencies transduced near the oval window and low frequencies near the apex of the cochlea. The output of the hair cells is conducted in the acoustic nerve to the cochlear nuclei from which second-order neurons cross and ascend in the contralateral lateral lemniscus. Some neurons project to the superior olive and others to the reticular formation bilaterally.

Hearing loss from a brainstem lesion is uncommon. Vestibular Schwannoma produces hearing loss often with tinnitus. Cortical damage can produce dysfunction of interpretation of auditory information, but this is the boundary between auditory abnormality and language abnormality.

When a patient presents with the report of hearing loss, the following information is key to diagnosis:

■ Is the deficit a problem with hearing threshold or loss of comprehension?
■ Is the deficit unilateral or bilateral?
■ Is there tinnitus?

Testing of hearing consists of:

■ hearing of speech
■ Weber and Rinne test
■ assessment of language comprehension.

Performance of Weber and Rinne tests is presented in Chapter 1. On the basis of information for history and examination, the following general rules apply:

■ Decreased hearing threshold suggests a cochlear or ear problem.
■ Bilateral hearing loss without other neurological signs is almost never due to neurological lesions.
■ Unilateral hearing loss with tinnitus raises concern about vestibular Schwannoma.
■ Bilateral tinnitus with hearing loss and vertigo with a waxing and waning course suggests Meniere's disease.

■ Decreased comprehension of verbal input with preserved hearing threshold suggests a retrocochlear (i.e. nerve or CNS) lesion.

Smell and taste

Smell is carried by the olfactory nerve, cranial nerve I. The sensory receptors are on small cells, the processes of which project through the cribiform plate.

Taste is carried mainly by the facial nerve to the brainstem, although a small amount of taste sensation from the posterior tongue is served by the glossopharyngeal (IX) nerve.

Taste and smell are considered together because they are interrelated in identification of food and deficits of one can be misinterpreted as deficit in the other. Taste determines the elemental content of the food: sweet, salt, bitter, sour. Smell adds detection of fine chemical analysis of the food. Only a few molecules are required to elicit an identification.

A patient with the inability to smell may complain of the inability to taste food, but formal testing shows that elemental taste is unaffected.

Important causes of loss of smell are:

■ head injury
■ sinus disease
■ toxins; sometimes strong odors can cause anosmia
■ neurodegenerative diseases, particularly Parkinsonism.

Important causes of loss of taste are:

■ facial palsy – though unlikely to be bilateral;
■ oropharyngeal tumors;
■ brainstem lesions, though unusual without other neurologic symptoms.

Taste and smell are not routinely tested, but if there is a specific complaint, then they should each be tested. For *smell*, blinded identification of coffee or chocolate is appropriate. Mint or smelling salts (ammonia) should not be used because these are trigeminal stimulants. For *taste*, sugar or salt should be blindly tested, although absolute inability to perceive these is extremely uncommon.

Pearls

- Numbness and tingling in the absence of pain or motor loss is seldom due to a serious condition.
- Most causes of numbness and tingling can be diagnosed by the distribution of the symptoms.
- Hearing loss without other symptoms or signs is rarely neurologic.
- Transient monocular blindness (amaurosis fugax) should be considered to be a TIA for evaluation and treatment.

When to refer

- When the cause of the sensory loss in unknown.
- When the identified cause requires expert neurological or neurosurgical care.
- When somatosensory symptoms do not respond to conventional therapy.

chapter 7

Pain

Approach to the patient

Pain is essentially an information system, which signals to us that there is something wrong, and the immediate requirement is to rectify or ameliorate the 'pathological' process causing the pain where possible. If this cannot be achieved, or the pain persists in spite of removal of the pathological process, the pain itself becomes the 'pathology' to be addressed. Allowing our patients to suffer 'pointless pain' is medical anathema anyway, but there are potentially severe secondary effects from continuing pain such as tissue atrophy, autonomic dysfunction and depression.

The first question is: What is the nature of the process causing the pain and what is its precise location? A detailed history is crucial to tease this out and a questionnaire can be an extremely helpful initial measure. The physical examination will then identify the exact location, and where doubt exists, a therapeutic trial can often help delineate the source, e.g. proton pump inhibitors relieve virtually all acid–pepsin related symptoms.

A great deal of general practice depends on identification, classification, and diagnosis of pain. In this chapter, we will discuss pain from a neurological standpoint – related more to etiology and treatment rather than specific cause. The classes of pain are:

- neuropathic pain
- musculoskeletal pain
- visceral pain
- headache.

Headache is discussed further in Chapter 3. Visceral pain seldom has a neurologic cause and is not considered here. Table 7.1 considers some general features of these different types of pain. Table 7.2 presents some of the medicines which we find helpful for treatment of pain.

Neuropathic pain

Neuropathic pain is generated directly in the nerves rather than being merely carried in the nerves after activation of nociceptive receptors. Repetitive action potentials produce a painful sensation. Therefore, treatment of neuropathic pain frequently relies on reduction in the repetitive action potentials.

Neurologists divide neuropathic pain into two general categories, *small fiber* and *large fiber*. Small fiber refers to small unmyelinated axons which carry pain and temperature sensation. Pain due to damage to these fibers is a burning or gnawing pain. Large fiber refers to the large diameter myelinated axons. Damage to these axons produces shooting or stabbing pain.

Treatment of small and large fiber neuropathic pain differs, in that tricyclic antidepressants are of greater use for the small-fiber pain whereas the anticonvulsants are of greater use for the large-fiber pain.

Diagnosis
Diagnosis of types of neuropathic pain is a clinical diagnosis but EMG, if available, can be supportive. If the EMG shows peripheral neuropathy, the diagnosis is secure; however, neuropathic pain may be present with a normal EMG if the affected nerve is not testable by routine EMG, or if the patient has a particular type of small-fiber

Table 7.1 Classification of pain syndromes

Type	Physiology	Causes	Treatment
Neuropathic – large fiber	Repetitive discharge of the large-diameter myelinated axons	Nerve trauma, herpes zoster, some peripheral neuropathies	Carbamazepine, gabapentin, baclofen, oxcarbazepine
Neuropathic – small fiber	Repetitive discharge of the small-diameter unmyelinated axons	Diabetes mellitus, amyloidosis, some toxins, some peripheral neuropathies	Amitriptyline, gabapentin, oxcarbazepine
Muscular	Inflammation of muscles stimulating pain nerves	Trauma, ischemia, inflammatory myopathy	Antiinflammatories. Muscle relaxants, if needed
Skeletal	Destruction or inflammation of periosteum and/or bone causing activation of pain fibers	Trauma, arthritis, tumor	Pure analgesics, anti-inflammatories
Visceral	Destruction or distention activating intrinsic pain fibers	Destructive lesion such as tumor, ischemia, distention	Pure analgesics, usually necessitates treating underlying cause

Table 7.2 Medications for pain

Generic name	Brand name	Supplied	Dose	Notes
Paracetamol Acetominophen	Paracetamol Tylenol	Tabs: 500 mg	2 tabs qid prn	
Nalbuphine	Nubain	Amps: 10 mg	10–20 mg i.m. or i.v. as needed	Agonist/antagonist, so can precipitate opiate withdrawal
Codeine and paracetamol	Tylex Tylenol 3	Paracetamol 500 mg, codeine 30 mg	1–2 q4h prn	
Oxycodone sustained release	Oxycontin	Tabs: 10, 20, 40, 80 mg	Start: 10 mg bid, increase as needed slowly	Only for moderate to severe pain. Special care for non-malignant pain
Morphine sustained release	Morcap SR MST Continus	Caps: 20, 50, 100 mg Tabs: 5, 10, 15, 30, 50, 100, 200 mg. Also available as liquid	20 q12h to start	

neuropathy, burning pain with distortion of hot–cold sensation can be prominent with normal EMG.

Treatment

Treatment of neuropathic pain is mainly accomplished with anti-epileptic drugs (AEDs), antidepressants, and analgesics. AEDs decrease the repetitive action potentials which cause the pain. Antidepressants (particularly the tricyclics) have a CNS effect in decreasing pain, but also help the depression which is usually coexistent with chronic neuropathic pain.

Anti-epileptic drugs (AEDs)

AEDs are the cornerstones of therapy for neuropathic pain. The most commonly used AEDs are:

- carbamazepine
- gabapentin
- lamotrigine
- oxcarbazepine.

Others are occasionally used, including phenytoin, valproate, and topiramate, although the evidence to support the effectiveness of these agents is less solid than the evidence for the listed agents.

Doses that are helpful for neuropathic pain are typically less than the doses required for the treatment of seizures.

AEDs are most effective for treatment of large-fiber neuropathic pain. This is the shooting, stinging pain. Gabapentin may also be effective for the small-fiber burning neuropathic pain.

Tricyclic antidepressants (TCAs)

TCAs are mainly helpful for the small fiber, burning neuropathic pain.

Amitriptyline and imipramine are usually used, although nortriptyline is also effective. The risk of cardiac conduction defects should be considered, and ECGs may be required.

The dose of TCAs for neuropathic pain is usually less than the dose required for depression. Amitriptyline doses of approximately 25 to 100 mg are typical, although in the elderly, starting dose of 10 mg would be appropriate.

Adverse effects have limited the use of TCAs for depression in the elderly, and the same is true for use in neuropathic pain. Exacerbation of dementia and confusion even in non-demented patients may occur, and there may be a hangover effect.

Pure analgesics
Pure analgesics are used as a rescue effort to give relief of neuropathic pain. In general, neuropathic pain does not respond as well as musculoskeletal pain to analgesics, but daily use may be helpful. Some patients only require medication at night. Therefore, an evening depropoxyphene may be sufficient.

It has been said by some that the abuse potential for the sustained-release formulations of opiate analgesics is low, but this is not uniformly true. It is prudent to try to avoid opiates in neuropathic (non-malignant) pain, but they are occasionally used in the short-term only with a good understanding between the physician and patient.

Capsaicin
Topical capsaicin is occasionally used for patients with neuropathic pain. Unfortunately, it can irritate the nerves when initially applied, and does not help many patients. Nevertheless, there are no central adverse effects, so it should be considered. It is important to warn the patient that initial exacerbation of symptoms may occur.

Musculoskeletal pain

Musculoskeletal pain is characterized by pain that originates from the contractile units (muscle, tendon, teno-periosteal junction, musculo-tendinous junctions) and from the non-contractile elements (joint, bursa, ligament, periosteum). If the contractile element is at fault, then the contraction of that unit against resistance will produce the pain, e.g. tennis elbow. If the pain originates from a non-contractile element, then the appropriate passive movement(s) will reproduce the pain. Palpation can then be used to localize the exact part of the inculpated structure and appropriate treatment initiated (e.g. localized steroid injection).

Evaluation

X-rays tend to be rather unhelpful in investigating these lesions, though any suspicion of primary bone disease (e.g. Paget's) or malignancy would mandate x-rays, blood tests and probably radionuclide imaging. Therefore, a therapeutic trial prior to performing many tests is warranted.

If there are findings on clinical presentation to suggest malignancy or other pathological causes of the pain, then plain x-rays are often performed along with radionuclide bone scan.

Treatment

Bone pain is typically treated by use of anti-inflammatory agents and pure analgesics. In general, there is little effective difference between the beneficial effects of the individual agents; however, there are greater differences between the adverse effects of the drugs. The newer COX-2 inhibitors have a lower incidence of gastrointestinal problems. For most patients, the routine NSAIDs are usually effective. These include:

- ibuprofen
- naproxen
- diclofenac
- indomethacin.

Important clinical presentations

A brief discussion of some of the common presenting pain syndromes may be illustrative.

Pain originating in the lumbar spine

Most pains in the lumbar region are caused by disc protrusions pressing on a nociceptive receptor rich structure. If the protrusion pressed on the dura mater alone, then the symptoms and signs will be:

- *Articular.* One, two or three of the four lumbar movements – flexion/extension/two side-flexions – will cause pain. Axiomatically a protrusion cannot cause pain in all four directions.
- *Dural.* A cough hurts by ballooning the venous sinuses against the disc, straight leg raise (SLR) is positive (this pulls on nerve roots L4–5, S1–2, moving the dura 2 to 5 mm over the displaced disc). Ely's Test is positive – prone-lying knee flexion pulls on the L3 root pulling on the dura and causing lumbar pain.

If the disc presses on the nerve root, then the pain becomes more severe and generally outlines the dermatome of the inculpated root. SLR or Ely's Test will pull on the trapped root, making the pain worse. Further pressure on the nerve root will lead to a neurological deficit in the corresponding territory.

If the evidence is purely of articular and dural pressure, manipulation of a solid fragment can be instantly curative. Root pain, with or without neurological deficit, means that manipulation will not help and blocking the pain route with epidural local anesthesia is appropriate. NSAIDs are potentially helpful at all stages, reducing inflammation at the site of the prolapse.

But what if disabling pain persists? The final decision on surgical intervention will rest with the surgeon himself, and his experience and philosophy. Willingness to intervene varies considerably, and the choice of surgeon is best directed by the physical and emotional needs of the patients. Appropriate referrals include:

- disturbance of sphincter control: mandatory and urgent!;
- radicular weakness refractory to conservative care;
- patient request for surgical opinion;
- intractable pain (i.e. refractory to conservative care).

This latter is a moot point. What constitutes intractable pain and what constitutes failed conservative care differs for individual clinicians. In general, patients should be counseled that:

- Surgery for pain alone is discouraged.
- Surgery for weakness does not improve the strength immediately. It allows the weakness to improve after the compression of the nerve root is resolved.
- Most patients with radiculopathy do not need surgery.

Only when the patient has clearly been apprised of the relative risks and benefits of surgery should referral be considered.

Pain blocks include epidural steroid injections, facet blocks, and selective root blocks. Each of these techniques has barely more than a 50% response rate and single treatments are seldom curative. Patients should understand that the blocks are helpful but do not cure the underlying condition.

Studies of treatment for back pain reinforce the view that there is no 'magic bullet'. When underlying causes of pain have been dealt with, the patient should be advised to do what has to be done in order to get on with his or her life.

Trigeminal neuralgia

Trigeminal neuralgia is characterized by episodes of severe lancinating pain in the distribution of one or more branches of the trigeminal nerve. One theory is that the pain is due to compression of the trigeminal nerve by a small vessel.

Chewing and eating often exacerbate the pain. Symptoms can come and go over years without known provoking or ameliorating factors.

Medical treatment for trigeminal neuralgia includes the following:

- carbamazepine
- gabapentin
- oxcarbazepine
- baclofen
- opiates.

Treatment typically begins with carbamazepine. If escalating doses are not effective, gabapentin or oxcarbazepine are used, roughly in that order.

Chronic opiates are seldom used in neurological patients with non-malignant pain, but they may be needed for limited periods in some patients. Try not to use opiates indefinitely, but rather while AEDs are being initiated. AEDs have been shown to be a good adjunct to opiates in this setting, since the dose of opiates required is lessened in the presence of especially carbamazepine or gabapentin.

Surgery is considered for patients with medically refractory trigeminal neuralgia. Happily, surgery is only performed on a small proportion of patients with trigeminal neuralgia. Among the surgeries available are:

- radiofrequency lesion (RFL)
- stereotactic radiosurgery
- microvascular decompression (the Janetta operation).

Stereotactic radiosurgery is becoming more popular over time, although its long-term efficacy has not been proved. This is a non-invasive technique which involves administration of high-energy photons delivered in a series of highly focused and precisely targeted arcs. The center of rotation of the arcs determines the area of highest intensity of the photons. The exposure of the remainder of the brain is negligible. If the equipment is functioning properly and the procedure performed competently, the technique is extremely safe and effective for most patients, at least in the short term.

Diabetic neuropathy

Diabetic neuropathy can be manifest as peripheral polyneuropathy, mononeuropathy multiplex, autonomic neuropathy, and simple mononeuropathy. Since diabetic neuropathy can produce small- and large-fiber pain, agents for both are typically used. Amitriptyline is used especially for the burning pain that keeps patients awake at night. Gabapentin is used especially for patients with shooting or stabbing pain, although this drug can help burning pain, as well. Gabapentin is used more than other AEDs largely because of its freedom from adverse effects and lack of drug interactions, a factor which is especially important in diabetic patients on multiple medications. Remember that gabapentin is excreted in the urine, so that renal insufficiency demands lower doses, especially initially, until the patient's tolerance can be determined.

At the present time, there is no cure for diabetic neuropathy or any neuropathy where there is not an identified reversible cause. There is a general impression that better control of the diabetes makes for better preservation of peripheral nerve function, but there is extreme variability among patients in glucose control and severity of neuropathy. Nerve growth factor is under investigation to determine whether it may promote regrowth of damaged nerve fibers in diabetics, but the studies are incomplete and, so far, unimpressive. A final decision on availability is likely two or more years away.

Post-herpetic neuralgia (PHN)

PHN is a severe pain syndrome that occurs after a breakout of herpes zoster. Current studies indicate that the incidence of PHN is lessened by treatment with acyclovir during an eruption. Dose of acyclovir is 800 mg five times daily for 7 days. Alternative treatment could be with famciclovir 500 mg t.i.d. for 7 days.

Recent data also suggests that the incidence of persistence of PHN is lessened by administration of amitriptyline 25 mg daily within 5 days of the onset of the symptoms.

Treatment of PHN is usually with:

- amitriptyline
- carbamazepine
- gabapentin

Chronic pain syndrome

Patients with chronic pain have impairment in their quality of life due to neurological and psychological manifestations of the pain. This is true for every pain condition from end-stage metastatic cancer to fibromyalgia. The relative balance between these pain divisions and the adaptation to them determines the real quality-of-life.

Neurological symptoms in chronic pain consist of the pain and other sensory disturbances related to activation of nociceptors and conduction through spino-thalamic tracts to the brain.

Pain perception can change over time in that there can be alteration in central pain conduction and in receptor fields. This activation produces facilitation in conduction to the brain which can enhance one's perception of pain. Also, the area of the body that is identified as having pain is increased in size due to alteration in the receptive fields.

Acute and chronic pain can inhibit muscle activity because of pathways that try to decrease worsening of an injury. This is termed antalgic weakness. In general, antalgic weakness is often thought by physicians to be psychosomatic, as maximal power and reflexes are normal, although anyone who has sustained a significant injury limiting muscle movement can testify to the real nature of the weakness. The body does not want to make a movement that hurts.

Psychological symptoms include the emotional reaction to the pain, inhibition of activity, and ultimately a dependency on the pain. The emotional reaction to the pain is more than sorrow about the experience, the patient's mood is changed. The incidence of depression is increased and patients often have a sense of anhedonia which is persistent. Inhibition of activity includes not only antalgic weakness but also apathy which decreases spontaneous movement.

Some particular psychological profiles come up regularly in intractable pain situations:

- Identification with someone (alive/dead/close/remote) who has a similar pain.
- Unbearable conflict issues in the person's life, where a decision either way would be extremely difficult and the pain spares them the pain of making the decision.
- Guilt.
- Imprint. In a situation of high stress, a patient can respond dramatically to a careless word or misunderstanding.

■ Purpose. The pain may well save the patient from unpleasant situations; e.g. backache saves them from going to their hated place of work. This is not true malingering, as the pain mechanisms are often subconscious.

Fibromyalgia

Fibromyalgia is destined to be one of the great non-diseases of our time. This opinion is certain to engender some disagreement from supporters of fibromyalgia as a distinct entity. However, the preponderance of data supports the notion that this is not a disease but a pain syndrome where multifocal pain and tenderness are the principal features. A few patients with fibromyalgia may have some undiagnosed connective tissue disease, and rare patients will be found to have peripheral neuropathy, but neuropathy does not typically produce fibromyalgia-like symptoms, so when it is identified in these patients, it is doubtful that the neuropathy is responsible for the fibromyalgia symptoms.

Clinical examination of patients with fibromyalgia consists of examination for strength and reflexes and sensory function as well as a survey for rash and joint deformity. Some of the conditions which should be considered in a patient being evaluated for fibromyalgia should include:

■ lupus
■ polymyalgia rheumatica
■ rheumatoid arthritis
■ neuropathy.

Once these and other organic conditions have been ruled-out as causing the patient's symptoms, treatment can begin. The treatment options are many, but one approach includes:

■ NSAIDs to treat a chronic arthritic or other inflammatory process which may have begun the process;
■ antidepressants which can help the patient's mood;
■ hypnotics if indicated;
■ exercise to stretch muscles and ligaments and gradually improve tolerance of activity.

Psychological consultation may be needed, but is not necessary for all patients. Having a sympathetic and listening doctor can be as helpful. If psychological consultation is needed, it can be presented to the patient as being for the purpose of helping the patient deal with their chronic condition rather than being presented as treatment of the psychological issues which perpetuate the disease process.

Chronic fatigue syndrome

Chronic fatigue syndrome is usually diagnosed as a disorder associated with fibromyalgia, and refers to the persistent fatigue which prevents the patients from engaging in normal family and occupational activities.

There are reports of biochemical abnormalities identified in patients with chronic fatigue syndrome, but these changes may be secondary to the disease process rather than primary, similar to the physiological changes seen in 'reflex sympathetic dystrophy', discussed below.

Chronic fatigue syndrome is best treated by:

- increased activity
- counseling about aggravating factors
- antidepressants.

Increased activity may take the form of structured physical therapy early in the course of the disease, but is then followed by involvement in a local health club. Counseling can be helpful to determine which factors may be precipitating the condition, such as job dissatisfaction, family pressures, etc. Bedtime TCAs can aid sleep in addition to having an antidepressant effect. SSRIs during the day can be helpful for increasing energy in addition to having an antidepressant effect.

Support groups are helpful for many chronic disorders, including Alzheimer's and stroke, but unfortunately, they may not be of help for patients with fibromyalgia and chronic fatigue syndrome, since they may produce a reinforcement for the patients which perpetuates the disorder and even expands the scope of symptoms as new manifestations are appreciated.

Complex regional pain syndromes

Reflex sympathetic dystrophy (RSD) is a disorder less diagnosed now than it once was. Most neurologists believe that RSD is neuropathic pain plus disuse atrophy. The origin of the neuropathic pain can be any insult, and the cause may be trivial. The scope and distribution of the pain may increase because of neurological and psychological factors discussed above. The patient stops using the affected extremity. This results in muscle wasting, skin changes, and bone changes which can all be reproduced in animals simply by the disuse without a neural lesion.

The key to treatment of RSD is prevention. If a patient with a neural injury can be returned to normal functioning and have the neuropathic pain promptly managed, the secondary disuse atrophy will not develop.

Causalgia is a term which has largely been discarded now, but refers to progressive pain, swelling, atrophy, and loss of use which occur after injury to a major nerve trunk. In contrast to RSD, there is initially a solid organic basis for the disuse, since movement in many patients can certainly exacerbate neuropathic pain. However, the degree of disuse and the scope of atrophy begin to extend far beyond the anatomic distribution of the nerve trunk damage. Treatment is essentially the same as for RSD, although there has to be aggressive treatment of the neuropathic pain so that function can be restored.

These conditions are now termed *complex regional pain syndrome*, with CRPS type I being RSD and CRPS type II being causalgia. This change in terminology accomplishes little other than emphasizing the relationship between these conditions.

When to refer

- Psychopathology which prevents the patient from responding well to treatment and returning to function in family and society – *psychology or psychiatry*

Pearls

- Bear in mind the psychosocial factors in chronic pain.
- Aim to control the pain for 24 hours a day – especially if opiates are deployed. This will tend to avoid dosage escalation and 'addiction'.
- Use TCAs for burning neuropathic pain.
- Use AEDs for shooting stinging neuropathic pain.

- Evidence of ongoing neural compression or infiltration – *Neurology or neurosurgery.*
- Regional blocks may be needed – *Pain clinics or anesthesiology.*

chapter 8

Seizures and other spells

Approach to the patient

The first task for the general physician when a seizure is suspected is to find out precisely what happened and the best way to do this is to ask witnesses for a verbal or (ideally) written account. The clear-cut case will usually fall into one of the following sorts:

- primary generalized tonic-clonic seizure;
- primary generalized 'absence' seizure;
- simple partial seizure;
- complex partial seizure; or
- not a seizure.

Simple means that there was no alteration of consciousness; *complex* means that there was an alteration of consciousness.

Partial means that there was a localized neurological symptom (numbness, weakness), or sign (e.g. motor activity such as lip smacking). The partial seizures may lead to a *generalized* seizure, i.e. a complex partial seizure with *secondary generalization.*

Primary generalized tonic-clonic seizure

The patient has sudden loss of consciousness, extension of the trunk and limbs often accompanied by 'the cry' and followed by the clonic phase of muscle jerking. He then goes through stupor to drowsy to confusion to sleepy but awake.

Primary generalized 'absence' seizure

Absence attacks begin in childhood and although they only last a few seconds can recur many times during the day and play havoc with the education of a perfectly normal child. These are staring spells during which time there may be some mouth movement, but the complex automatic movements of complex partial seizures are usually absent. Also, the patient returns immediately to their pre-ictal activities, in contrast to complex partial seizures which disrupt the thought process.

Many children with absence epilepsy will also have generalized tonic-clonic seizures. When these new seizures develop, this is not a sign of new neuropathology, and does not necessarily mean that repeat EEG/scan study is needed.

The EEGs of patients with absence epilepsy are usually abnormal, in contrast to many other forms of seizure where an EEG may be normal in the inter-ictal period.

Simple partial seizure

The patient has a focal seizure that does not proceed to generalization. The seizure is focal motor or sensory and does not disturb consciousness. If the seizure spreads to other areas of the brain, producing a generalized seizure, this is termed a secondary generalized seizure, as opposed to the primary generalized seizure that does not have a cortical focus.

Complex partial seizure

A complex partial seizure has a focal origin but the locus is such that consciousness is typically affected. The hallmark is stereotypism – it is usually the same every time, e.g. lip smacking, dejà vu, olfactory sensation. Identifying the partial onset may be difficult since the patient will usually have no recollection of the event. The term complex refers to the fact that mental status is affected, disturbing the patient's ability to interact with the environment.

The location is most commonly in the temporal lobe, although extra-temporal locations can also be present, e.g. frontal lobe. The EEG will usually show the focal onset and often shows inter-ictal focal spiking. One cannot distinguish temporal from frontal lobe foci on clinical grounds alone. These used to be called 'temporal lobe' or 'psychomotor' seizures.

Secondary generalized seizure

This is a generalized seizure, usually tonic-clonic, which has a partial onset. Identifying the partial onset may be difficult since the patient will usually have no recollection of the event. Also, observers may not identify the partial symptoms at the onset, e.g. lip smacking. The EEG will usually show the focal onset and often shows inter-ictal focal spiking.

Table 8.1 summarizes features of different seizure types.

Evaluation

Epilepsy is defined as repeated unprovoked seizures. Every epileptic patient should have the benefit of a neurological opinion. However, the general physician referral letter needs to indicate the urgency of the consultation by noting the severity of the attack, frequency of recurrences, and the anxiety level in the patient or relatives and whether AEDs has been initiated. If the attack was atypical and the diagnosis in doubt, this should also be noted.

Most patients with new-onset seizures should be subject to the following investigations:

- Brain imaging (preferably MRI with and without contrast enhancement)
- complete blood cell count (CBC) and metabolic panel
- drug screen
- EEG.

MRI is the preferred mode of imaging for patients with partial seizures. Low-grade tumors and other infiltrating lesions may not be seen on CT.

Table 8.1 Classification of seizures

Type	Clinical features	EEG findings	Treatment
Primary generalized tonic-clonic	Sudden loss of consciousness, fall, shaking and stiffening of the extremities	Bursts of spike and slow wave complexes with the seizures and often between clinical seizures, as well	Phenytoin, valproate, clonazepam
Primary generalized absence	Staring spells without warning. May be subtle mouth movements	Bursts of 3-per-second spike and wave complexes during and between seizures. Worse with hyperventilation	Ethosuximide, valproate
Simple partial	Shaking of one extremity or one side of the body	Focal spike activity over one hemisphere, usually in the central region	Phenytoin, carbamazepine
Complex partial	Various forms. Disturbance of consciousness though may appear awake. Stereotypic movements of the limbs and/or mouth	Normal or focal slow activity or spikes in a temporal or frontal distribution	Carbamazepine, phenytoin, oxcarbazepine, levetiracetam
Myoclonic	Episodes of brief jerks of inappropriate relations of the limbs without disturbance of consciousness	Normal or may show a burst of spikes with the episodes	Valproate, clonazepam, levetiracetam

Please note: other treatments are effective but the drugs listed are of special importance.

CBC is performed to look for signs of infection, although some chronic CNS infections may have no systemic laboratory findings. A metabolic panel is done to look for renal and hepatic dysfunction, not only because these disorders could lower seizure threshold, but also because even incipient renal or hepatic dysfunction could influence drug selection for the seizures.

An EEG is performed to characterize the seizure discharges. In some instances this can guide proper drug selection. For example, very different drugs are used for a patient with staring spells if the EEG shows a 3-per-second spike-wave pattern (absence epilepsy) or a focal right temporal discharge (complex partial epilepsy).

Treatment while awaiting neurological opinion

A single generalized tonic-clonic seizure does not always warrant medication. With a single unprovoked seizure in an adult, the rate of recurrence varies between 30 and 70% in various studies. Armed with this information, some patients elect to not take medicine, essentially taking their chances that they will not have another seizure. Of course, typical seizure precautions apply, including not driving, operating dangerous machinery, or otherwise engaging in activities which could endanger them or others if they were to have a seizure.

For many patients, treatment cannot await neurological consultation. Initial treatments for the types of seizures are discussed in Table 8.1. In general, phenytoin or carbamazepine is usually used for primary generalized tonic-clonic seizures. Ethosuximide is used first for absence epilepsy, although valproate is an alternative. Carbamazepine is usually used first for partial seizures.

Absence attacks recur so frequently that treatment is usually essential. Benign rolandic epilepsy, a specific type of partial-onset seizure in children, often does not require treatment.

Valproate is one of the most powerful medicines available for seizure treatment, although its use is limited because of some safety concerns. Care should especially be exercised in women of childbearing potential, as the rate of fetal malformations, particularly neural-tube defects, is increased in exposed fetuses. Valproic acid also may cause hair loss, weight gain and menstrual irregularities, all of which render it less than ideal in young women. Also, there is concern over hepatotoxicity, particularly in young children, and in patients on multiple anticonvulsants. This risk is extremely low in adults, especially over 30 years of age.

Some general points on management

- Most patients should be managed with a single drug, monitoring blood levels as needed to maintain the patient seizure free. They should initially have a 3-monthly and then a yearly blood test to screen out the uncommon toxicities (e.g. blood dyscrasias, macrocytosis, hyponatremia).
- The specialist epilepsy nurse is developing a growing role in advising, counseling and day-to-day management of these conditions.
- Difficult cases may need to be reviewed frequently by the neurologist and 'open-access' is often appropriate.
- Consistency of advice is vital, the physician should choose a neurologist whose opinion is respected, who is easy to speak to and with whom the physician has a good relationship.
- Warn all patients about potential for adverse effects of the anticonvulsants, and give some general guidance on how to deal with these symptoms.
- Patients who may have seizures (or any other condition characterized by loss of consciousness) should not operate motor vehicles, operate dangerous machinery, swim alone or work at unprotected heights.

Epilepsy mimics and related conditions

'Aggravated' syncope
Feeling faint resolves itself naturally by the fall to the ground which restores perfusion to the brain. However, if the patient

maintains a seated position the cerebral hypoxia may lead to a seizure indistinguishable from true epilepsy. However, a careful history of the pre-'ictal' events should distinguish the two. This is sometimes called clonic or convulsive syncope. This should not be treated with AEDs, if the diagnosis is secure.

Stokes–Adams attacks

An older person falls to the floor with sinus arrest, going pale and then gray, and, as in aggravated syncope, the cerebral hypoxia can trigger seizures before normal blood pressure is restored.

These would be the archetypes of the various cardiovascular causes of cerebral hypoxia leading to seizures.

Migraine

Rarely migraine with aura may be difficult to distinguish from simple partial seizure. A careful history should tease out the longer duration of the migraine aura and its typical features. Bear in mind that seizures and migraines may co-exist in the same patient.

Transient ischemic attacks

TIAs can occasionally be mistaken for seizures. The cerebral anoxia may trigger some trembling or jerking along with the transient neurological deficit (the shaking TIA often related to carotid stenosis). Fortunately, careful history and observation can usually make the distinction. EEG may still be necessary, however. Much more rare are focal seizures which produce transient paralysis without any positive motor activity. Only EEG can distinguish this from TIA; however, multiple events over a long period of time, which are refractory to antiplatelet agents, suggests this diagnosis.

Hypoglycemia

Usually there will be pronounced autonomic accompaniments to the hypoglycemic symptoms (e.g. sweating, palpitations) but neurological symptoms and signs may predominate. Patients with long-standing diabetes with autonomic neuropathy commonly fail to have the adrenergic symptoms associated with hypoglycemia.

Sleep disorders

Narcolepsy can occasionally be confused with epilepsy, as patients have the uncontrollable urge to lie down and sleep. These episodes occur in attacks, so they may be thought of as being 'seizures' by the patient or family. A careful history is usually helpful for differentiation. Patients go to sleep and not into some other form of loss of consciousness.

Cataplectic attacks may also be confused with seizures in occasional patients, although this is not common.

Panic attacks

Panic attacks may present with funny feelings followed by dizziness. This is usually easy to distinguish from epilepsy, however, when coexistent hyperventilation results in tetany and syncope, the diagnosis is more in doubt. The typical clinical accompaniments of tachypnea, tachycardia, flushes and sweats with the sensation of suffocation, de-realization and fear of death should help to tease it out.

Psychogenic seizures

The GP will know the family background as a pointer, but these are the most difficult to distinguish, often requiring the simultaneous use of an EEG and video records. Some general features, which suggest pseudoseizures, include:

- Seizures only when family or friends are around.
- Triggering of seizures by stressful events.
- Failure of the seizures to respond to any anticonvulsant.
- Evidence of responsiveness on examination during a seizure, e.g. eyes roll up and away from the examiner when lids are held open; patient exactly opposes any passive movement of their limbs by the examiner; patient can be encouraged to communicate with eye-blinks during a seizure.
- Patient has multiple seizures per day until the EEG leads are placed, after which none are seen.

Drug treatment of epilepsy

There has been an explosion in the number of drugs for treatment of epilepsy. Most of these have been approved for add-on (adjunctive) therapy for partial seizures. However, this approval is a by-product of the methods of drug development. Studies are performed on patients with refractory seizures, which tend to be partial. Also, it would not be ethical to have a placebo-controlled trial of drugs used as monotherapy, so the drugs are tried as add-ons. In reality, the clinical utility of the drugs extends beyond partial seizures, and many of these are effective as monotherapy.

Adverse effects are common with use of these drugs. One could not find many drugs in the physician's Desk Reference that did not cause nausea, dizziness, or sedation. The incidence of these effects resulting in a call to the clinic is probably decreased rather than increased by warning the patient. If the effects are mild, they will probably pass, and only reassurance is needed. If the effects are severe, then the patient should be changed to another drug.

First-generation drugs

These are the 'old' drugs. The agents are listed in alphabetical order by generic name and tabulated in Table 8.2.

Carbamazepine

CBZ was first approved for use in trigeminal neuralgia, but has since been found to be effective for seizures. CBZ is frequently used first for complex partial seizures, especially in females and children for generalized seizures, except absence.

Blood monitoring is performed because of a risk of leukopenia, but this risk is fairly low, and the routine monitoring does not prevent the leukopenia from occurring.

Sustained-release versions of CBZ should be used, when available, because there is much greater compliance with b.i.d. dosing than t.i.d. or q.i.d. dosing. The half-life of the drug precludes b.i.d. dosing for this drug once auto-induction has taken place.

Table 8.2 Anticonvulsants – old drugs

Generic name	Brand name	Supplied	Dose	Note
Carbamazepine	Tegretol, Teril (USA: Epitol)	Tabs: 200 mg. Chew 100 mg. SR 100, 200, 300, 400 mg. Susp 100 mg/5 ml	Start: 200 mg bid, lower doses may be needed initially. Adjust dose to levels	Autoinduction after starting results in an initial sag in levels
Clonazepam	Rivotril	Tabs: 0.5, 2 mg	Start 0.5 mg bid. Taper slowly. Max 6 mg/day	IV formulation available for status or NPO use
Ethosuximide	Zarontin	Cap: 250 mg. Syrup: 250 mg/5 ml	Start: 250 mg bid, max 2000 mg/d. Adjust to levels	
Phenobarbital	Phenobarbitone	Tabs: 30, 60 mg. Elixir: 15 mg/5 ml	Start 30 mg qhs, max 180 mg qhs. Children 8 mg/kg/d	
Phenytoin	Epanutin (USA: Dilantin)	Caps: 30, 100 mg. Tabs: 50 mg. Susp: 125 mg/5 ml	Start: 100 mg tid. May be given as a single daily dose	Adjust to levels
Primidone	Mysoline	Tabs: 250 mg	Start: 125 mg qhs to usually 1 g/day max	Adjust to levels
Valproate	Convulex, Epilim, Depakote	Multiple formulations and strengths	Start: 125–250 mg bid. Children: 15 mg/kg/d to start, 30 mg/kg/d max in divided doses	Adjust to levels. Risk of birth defects, liver failure

Ethosuximide

Ethosuximide is used only for absence seizures. Some patients with mixed tonic-clonic plus absence seizures will have control with this agent, but valproate is commonly needed for these patients.

Phenobarbital (PB)

Phenobarbital is seldom used nowadays except in very young patients. Infants with seizures often have to be treated with it because phenytoin and other drugs are not absorbed well.

Phenytoin

Phenytoin continues to be a widely used drug for generalized and partial seizures, but is not used for absence seizures. There is a small risk of hematological toxicity, but not enough to require frequent CBC monitoring. Ataxia has been reported in some patients, who were treated with phenytoin for many years; however, with the widespread use of drug levels, this effect is less likely.

Birth defects are more likely in children of women with epilepsy and one of the offending agents may be phenytoin. A constellation of abnormalities has been termed the 'fetal hydantoin syndrome'. However, this constellation is not unique to phenytoin, looking much like the fetal alcohol syndrome and a number of others.

Primidone

Primidone is used for generalized and partial seizures. It is metabolized to an active metabolite, phenylethyl-malonamide (PEMA), plus PB. Therefore, levels of primidone and phenobarbital are usually checked simultaneously.

Sedative effects of primidone preclude its widespread use nowadays. However, there will be occasional patients with partial seizures who will respond to primidone when they do not respond to other agents. Primidone is presently used more for essential tremor than for seizures.

Valproate

Valproate is a powerful anticonvulsant, which is used for a broad range of seizure types including generalized tonic-clonic, absence, partial, and others.

Hepatic failure develops in a very small proportion of patients, necessitating blood monitoring. The risk of hepatic failure is greatest in younger patients and in patients on multiple anticonvulsants.

Teratogenicity limits the use of valproate in women of childbearing potential. All epileptics who have the potential for getting pregnant should be on folate, which reduces this risk. Patients on valproate should be strongly considered for other medications if they might get pregnant. This issue is one potential reason for neurological consultation.

Second-generation drugs

These drugs are much newer than the first-generation drugs. They have been developed largely for add-on therapy for partial seizures, although they are helpful for more than this. Most of these agents have a good safety profile, with the notable exception of the first, felbamate. These drugs are summarized in Table 8.3.

Felbamate

Felbamate is an extremely powerful anticonvulsant, but its use has been curtailed by the possibility of toxicity. Aplastic anemia or hepatic failure developed in a small number of patients, but the proportion was considered great enough that felbamate is now relegated to last-line treatment for most seizure types. Because of this precaution, most patients so-treated have had partial seizures. Frequent blood monitoring is required. Because of these concerns, only neurologists should prescribe felbamate.

Gabapentin

Gabapentin is used for patients with partial seizures, although there is evidence that it can be effective for generalized seizures as well. Gabapentin and levetiracetam have the lowest rates of drug–drug

Table 8.3 Anticonvulsants – new agents

Generic name	Brand name	Supplied	Dose	Note
Felbamate	Felbatol	Tabs: 400, 600 mg. Susp 600 mg/5 ml	Start: 400 mg tid. Max 1200 mg tid	Blood monitoring required
Gabapentin	Neurontin	Caps: 100, 300, 400 mg. Tabs: 600, 800 mg	Start: 300 mg tid. Max 1200 mg tid	If on VPA: start at 25 mg qod × 2 wk then 25 mg daily. Max 200 mg/day
Lamotrigine	Lamictal	Tabs: 25, 100, 150, 200 mg. Chew: 5, 25 mg	If no VPA: start at 25 bid. Taper: to 50 mg bid after 2 wk. Max 500 mg/day	
Levetiracetam	Keppra	Tabs: 500, 750 mg	Start: 500 mg bid. Taper: 250–500 mg/wk. Max 1500 mg bid	
Oxcarbazepine	Trileptal	Tabs: 150, 300, 600 mg	Start: 150 mg bid. Taper: 300 mg/d/wk, Max 600 mg bid	
Tiagabine	Gabitril	Tabs: 4, 12, 16, 20 mg	Start: 4 mg qam. Taper: 4 mg/d/wk. Max 32 mg/day	Patients on enzyme-inducing drugs require up to 56 mg/day
Topiramate	Topamax	Tabs: 25, 100, 200 mg	Start: 50 mg/day. Max 200 mg bid	
Zonisamide; not available in UK at time of publication	Zonegran	Caps: 100 mg	Start: 100 mg qam. Taper: 100 mg/wk. Max 400 mg/day	Small risk of urolithiasis

interactions, so these two are especially useful for patients on multiple other drugs. This feature also makes it especially suited to elderly patients.

The dose of gabapentin must be pushed up for good benefit; doses of 2400–3600 mg/day are usually required for good seizure control.

Gabapentin is used more for neuropathic pain than seizures, and is effective for both.

Lamotrigine

Lamotrigine is another powerful anticonvulsant that has a very broad spectrum of clinical use. Its main use is in refractory partial seizures, but since release it has been found to be useful in a number of other seizure types, including some childhood epilepsies. Absence seizures and the Lennox–Gastaut syndrome often respond to lamotrigine.

The risk of rash requires a slow tapering of dosage. Therefore, some weeks pass before good therapeutic doses may be administered. The dosing depends on whether the patient is on valproate, and the package insert should be followed to the letter, without acceleration of the rate of titration. In fact, some patients require an even slower rate of titration. No blood monitoring is required.

Levetiracetam

Levetiracetam is a new powerful anticonvulsant that was approved for add-on therapy of partial seizures but has since been found to be effective for patients with generalized tonic-clonic and myoclonic seizures. Starting doses are effective, although if there is not an adequate response, increasing the dose is essential. No blood monitoring is required.

Oxcarbazepine

Oxcarbazepine is chemically similar to carbamazepine (CBZ) and has a similar therapeutic profile. It is effective for partial seizures and generalized seizures and is also helpful for neuropathic pain.

No hepatic or hematological toxicity has been described with oxcarbazepine, so routine blood monitoring is not needed. As with any new drug, one should be sensitive to adverse effects, though. Occasional patients have developed hyponatremia, so routine blood monitoring is recommended.

Tiagabine

Tiagabine is approved for use in partial seizures. The risk of adverse effects is low, however, there is a small risk of encephalopathy. This possibility should be considered with epilepsy patients who present with mental status changes.

Topiramate

Topiramate is a new AED that is approved for partial seizures but likely has a wider clinical use. Being a carbonic anhydrase inhibitor, there is a small risk of urolithiasis, and patients should be warned about the potential symptoms which may suggest this. Topiramate can also cause confusion, which may be subtle. In contrast to most AEDs, it is more likely to cause weight loss than weight gain.

Zonisamide

Zonisamide is used for partial seizures and may be used as mono-therapy. It has a very long half-life and can be given once per day, which is a major boon to compliance. There is some weak carbonic anhydrase activity, but this seldom poses a problem.

Selection of agents for seizure types

Recommended treatment for the following seizure types can be insti-tuted by the generalist. Patients with other seizure types should be referred to a neurologist for consultation.

The physician's selection of drugs is like a soldier wearing an ammunition belt. There are only so many different types of ammuni-tion and weapons which can be carried on the belt. So, for the usual combatant, it is most prudent for the physician to load his or her belt with a selection of drugs that are safe, easy to use, and have a broad spectrum of action. For the general physician, one combination of weapons might be:

- phenytoin
- carbamazepine
- valproate
- ethosuximide
- levetiracetam.

Most of the other second-generation agents should be left to the neurologist. He or she will have discarded the first three weapons from his armamentarium, because they have already been tried in all referred patients.

Generalized tonic-clonic seizures
The drugs of choice for generalized tonic-clonic seizures are:

- phenytoin
- carbamazepine
- valproate.

Absence seizures
Absence epilepsy is most commonly treated with ethosuximide. Some patients with mixed absence and generalized tonic-clonic seizures will respond to ethosuximide although many of these patients will require valproate. Lamotrigine is an alternative which will may be used more widely in the future.

Simple partial seizures
First-line drugs for simple partial seizures usually are phenytoin and carbamazepine. One drug is first used as monotherapy. If good therapeutic levels are not effective in complete control of the seizures, then the other drug is used. There is less consensus on which drugs to use if these are ineffective. Most commonly, one of the second-generation drugs is used as add-on therapy. If this results in complete control, then the older drug may be slowly withdrawn to allow monotherapy with a single agent. While the new drugs are not widely approved for use as monotherapy, there is early evidence from small

studies and clinical practice to indicate that they are effective as monotherapy.

Complex partial seizures

Complex partial seizures are usually treated with carbamazepine, as first-line therapy, although phenytoin is a good alternative. Many feel that oxcarbazepine may eventually be shown to be just as effective as carbamazepine but with fewer adverse effects, but data on this are still incomplete. If a patient does not respond to carbamazepine, phenytoin or valproate may be used. Many of the new AEDs have a long track record of use in patients with complex partial seizures. Of the newer drugs, some of the most helpful ones are:

- lamotrigine
- levetiracetam
- topiramate
- oxcarbazepine
- zonisamide.

Gabapentin and tiagabine are both helpful for some patients, although these drugs are felt to be generally less effective than some of the other new ones.

Special populations of patients

Pregnancy

Women with epilepsy have an increased incidence of birth defects. AEDs increase this risk further. Unfortunately, the exact rate of birth defects with each of the agents is not known. Studies are currently underway to define this risk more clearly. Presently, the best estimation of risk from clinical trials and theoretical arguments suggests that the main drugs to be avoided during pregnancy are valproate, carbamazepine, topiramate, and zonisamide. By the time a woman knows she is pregnant, the early fetal stages of development are well underway, and many of the serious defects would have already occurred. Because of this and the frequency of unplanned pregnancies, it is recommended to avoid the use of these in women who are or have a reasonable likelihood of becoming pregnant.

Multiple concurrent medications

Concurrent medications result in drug interactions including binding changes, alterations in protein binding, renal clearance, and hepatic metabolism. For patients on few medications, this is usually not a major concern. For patients on multiple medications, gabapentin and levetiracetam have the lowest rate of drug interactions.

Oral contraceptives

Carbamazepine and oxcarbazepine are especially likely to make oral contraceptives less effective. The failure rate increases from perhaps 1% to 3–4%. Therefore, all women who are using oral contraceptive pills should be counseled about this effect, and should be considered for higher doses, and even consider an alternative method of birth control.

Surgical treatment of epilepsy

Surgical treatment of epilepsy has improved in the past few years. Patients who should be considered for referral for epilepsy surgery should meet the following criteria:

- Patient has refractory seizures.
- Patient has the ability to understand the implications of epilepsy surgery (i.e. patients who are not competent to make decisions will usually not be candidates for surgery).
- Patient is free of diseases that might shorten life expectancy, thereby making the patient less able to benefit from the procedure.

Pearls

- Tonic-clonic seizures with intact consciousness are usually pseudoseizures.
- Valproate should be avoided in women of childbearing potential.
- Labeling a patient an 'epileptic' has a great impact on his future, and should be used only when seizures recur; in the interim, the term seizure is appropriate.
- EEGs may be helpful, but the diagnosis remains clinical, with the accurate eyewitness account or video monitoring yielding the best evidence.
- Most patients (70%) can be controlled with a single drug with dose adjustment aided by blood levels.
- Self-help groups and epilepsy associations are useful to help the epileptic make the most of life with this diagnosis.
- Epileptics have a higher rate of fetal abnormality – up to 4× the normal population. Therefore screen in the first trimester with ultrasound and alpha-fetoprotein, so that a therapeutic termination may be offered.

When to refer

The vast majority of patients with seizures respond very well to medical treatment. Monotherapy suffices for most patients. However, the long-term implications to the patient are potentially so profound, that all patients with seizures should have at least one consultation with an expert. Further consultation may be advised when:

- seizures are imperfectly controlled;
- neurological signs/symptoms develop;
- seizure type changes.

chapter 9

Stroke and transient ischemic attack

Stroke is a sudden or rapid episode of brain injury with a vascular cause. It may produce a neurological deficit from pathology within a supplying artery, or symptoms from bleeding in and around the brain substance.

Transient ischemic attack (TIA) is a temporary neurological deficit due to interruption of blood flow. TIAs are always ischemic whereas strokes can be ischemic or hemorrhagic.

Approach to the patient

The key to identification of stroke and TIA is suspicion. The most common symptoms that could be stroke and TIA are:

- hemiparesis or hemisensory loss
- aphasia
- dysarthria
- diplopia
- unilateral visual loss – one eye or one hemifield
- abrupt onset of unusual headache.

Symptoms that are usually **not** stroke or TIA include:

- vertigo without other symptoms or signs
- syncope

- presyncopal sensations
- blurred vision.

In evaluating a stroke or TIA, the general physician's task is mainly to answer the following questions:

- how quickly does the patient need hospital referral?
- what sort of referral does he or she need?
- what needs to be done in the interim?
- what needs to be done to prevent recurrence?

Neurology referral is needed for acute stroke. Urgent CT is needed with new abrupt onset of headache, even without neurological deficit, or acute onset of any neurological deficit which could be vascular.

TIA can be evaluated as an outpatient as long as treatment is initiated. These issues are discussed in detail below.

Etiology of vascular disease

There are three principal mechanisms of stroke:

- thrombotic ischemic stroke
- embolic ischemic stroke
- hemorrhage.

Thrombotic stroke is due to atherosclerosis and/or arteriolar sclerosis (lipohyalinosis) that develops over the patient's life. This is the most common cause, responsible for one half of strokes.

Embolic stroke is commonly due to intracardiac thrombus formation and associated with atrial fibrillation and myocardial hypokinesis. Paradoxical embolization through a patent foramen ovale, aortic atherothrombi, and endocarditis (infective or non-infective) are less frequent sources of cerebral emboli. This is responsible for about a quarter of strokes.

Hemorrhage is due to rupture of the arteries, venous occlusions, blood dyscrasias, and amyloid deposition. Damage to the vessels from hypertension (arteriolar sclerosis) is the most important predisposing factor. There can also be a developmental abnormality in the vessel wall which predisposes to this. Hemorrhage accounts for 16% of strokes, with 6% being subarachnoid hemorrhage ((from berry aneurysm and vascular malformation rupture) and 10% intracerebral hemorrhage (from arteriosclerosis, blood dyscrasia, or amyloid angiopathy).

TIA is due to temporary ischemia and is usually related to small emboli from the large vessels and/or flow decrement across critically stenosed vessels. The emboli may lodge at a bifurcation of vessels

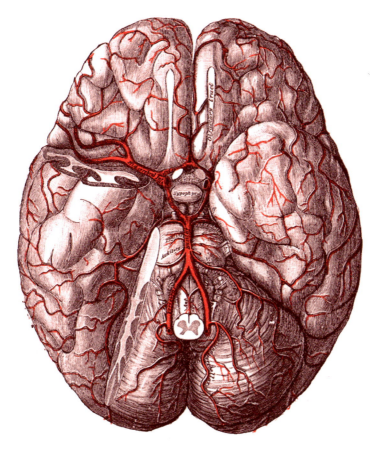

Figure 9.1 *Arterial supply to the brain. Reprinted from* Gray's Anatomy, *38th edn, Peter Williams (ed), 1995, by permission of the publisher Churchill Livingstone.*

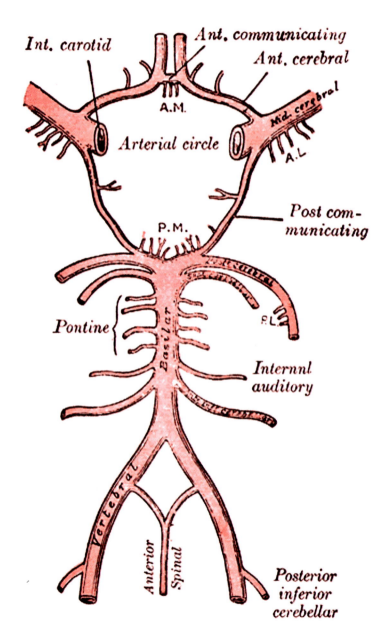

Figure 9.2 *Arterial supply to the brain. Reprinted from Gray's Anatomy, 38th edn, Peter Williams (ed), 1995, by permission of the publisher Churchill Livingstone.*

temporarily producing low flow. After a short time, pressure behind the embolus breaks it up and flow is restored (Figs 9.1 and 9.2).

Ischemic stroke syndromes

Most strokes and TIAs fall into a vascular territory, and the symptoms and signs indicate which vascular territory has been affected. If successive strokes or TIAs affect two different vascular territories, then proximal emboli are suspected. If the same vessel territory is affected each time, then damage to one vessel is suspected. Table 9.1 presents some key features of important stroke syndromes.

Anterior cerebral artery (ACA)

ACA strokes produce contralateral leg weakness. There may be arm weakness, but this is much less prominent than the leg weakness, and tends to involve proximal muscles (shoulder and upper arm) rather than distal muscles (hand).

ACA strokes are usually due to cerebral embolism. Most patients have hypertension and/or diabetes. This is less common than middle cerebral artery strokes.

The ACAs to both sides may have a common origin, so infarction can potentially produce bilateral leg weakness which can be mistaken for spinal cord lesion. Sphincter disturbance is even possible.

Middle cerebral artery (MCA)

This is the most common stroke syndrome. The reason for the prevalence is thought to be the 'straight-shot' in blood flow from the internal carotid artery to the MCA. Therefore, emboli from the carotid or the heart are likely to lodge in branches of the MCA.

MCA strokes produce contralateral weakness which affects the arm and face more than the leg and affects the distal arm muscles more than the proximal ones. MCA distribution infarction may develop from local vessel damage or to emboli from either the large proximal vessels or heart.

137

Table 9.1 Stroke syndromes

Vessel	Clinical findings
Infarction	
Anterior cerebral artery	Unilateral or bilateral leg weakness without arm deficits
Middle cerebral artery	Contralateral hemiparesis, arm greater than leg
Dominant hemisphere	Contralateral hemiparesis with aphasia
Non-dominant hemisphere	Contralateral hemiparesis with neglect
Posterior cerebral artery	Contralateral hemianopia and memory loss
Basilar artery	Crossed weakness or quadriparesis, often with diplopia, nausea, vomiting
Vertebral artery	Ataxia and weakness often with vertigo, nausea, diplopia
Lacunar infarct – lenticulostriate	Contralateral weakness and incoordination without aphasia, neglect, or other cortical signs
Lacunar infarct – thalamoperforate	Contralateral sensory loss, often with dysesthesias
Hemorrhage	
Subarachnoid hemorrhage	Abrupt onset of severe headache often with disturbance of consciousness
Hypertensive hemorrhage	Acute or subacute onset of weakness or ataxia, often with headache and confusion
Subdural hematoma	Subacute onset of weakness sometimes with seizures. May have headache, but not invariable
Epidural hematoma	Rapidly-progressive obtundation in the setting of recent trauma

138

In addition to weakness, cortical deficits are present. Of these findings, aphasia indicates a dominant (usually left) hemisphere stroke while neglect indicates a non-dominant (usually right) hemisphere stroke. About 50% of patients who are left-handed will still have the left hemisphere dominant for speech.

Posterior cerebral artery (PCA)

PCA infarcts produces visual loss which differs substantially from lesions affecting the anterior visual pathways. PCA infarct produces hemianopia or quadrantanopia. The superior or inferior quadrant may be affected. Cortical infarcts produce visual loss of which the patient is often unaware. Unlike lesions of the anterior visual pathways where the patient complains of a specific area of loss of vision, cortical lesions result in either unnoticed visual loss or a vague sense of something not being right about the vision. Hemianopia is the most likely significant localizing sign to be missed on neurological examination done by a non-expert.

The PCA supplies not only the occipital cortex but also the thalamus and medial temporal lobes. Therefore, contralateral sensory loss or memory loss may be seen with PCA infarction. The memory deficit usually improves substantially.

Because of the common origin of the PCAs from the basilar artery, bilateral PCA infarctions may occur, which then results in cortical blindness. The patient may complain of some non-specific visual difficulty, but otherwise, is frequently not totally aware of the deficit.

Vertebral and basilar arteries

The vertebral arteries join to form the basilar artery at the level of the caudal pons. The vertebral and basilar arteries supply the entirety of the brainstem and cerebellum.

Table 9.2 shows some of the most common brainstem syndromes.

Vertebral occlusion

Vertebral occlusion usually causes the lateral medullary syndrome. This is normally produced by occlusion of the posterior–inferior cerebellar artery (PICA) which is the most important intracranial

Table 9.2 Brainstem stroke syndromes

Syndrome	Cause	Features
Top-of-the-basilar syndrome	Embolus to the bifurcation of the basilar into the posterior cerebral arteries. Damage to midbrain, occipital lobes, medial temporal lobes	Cortical blindness, complex ocular motor defects, corticospinal signs, memory loss, sensory defects
Lateral medullary syndrome	Occlusion of the posterior inferior cerebellar artery or vertebral artery	Ipsilateral ataxia, Horner's syndrome, vertigo, contralateral loss of pain and temperature sense, ipsilateral loss of facial sense
Clumsy-hand dysarthria syndrome	Occlusion of a penetrating branch of the basilar artery in the pons	Hemiparesis, dysarthria, often with facial weakness
Pontine hemorrhage	Hypertensive hemorrhage of one of the penetrating branches of the basilar artery	Coma, quadriparesis with dysarthria, dysphagia, ataxia

branch of the vertebral artery. The PICA and the anterior spinal arteries are the major branches that arise from the vertebral artery but as the anterior spinal arteries are paired, spinal cord infarction does not result from a vertebral artery occlusion.

Occlusion of the PICA results in the lateral medullary syndrome, or Wallenberg's syndrome. The PICA supplies the lateral aspect of the medulla and occlusion results in ipsilateral Horner's syndrome, ipsilateral limb ataxia, ipsilateral loss of facial sensation, and contralateral loss of body pain and temperature sensation. Hoarseness is also common because of weakness of one vocal cord.

Basilar occlusion

Infarctions affecting the basilar artery territory may be produced by occlusion of the entire basilar artery or occlusion of one of the branches of the basilar artery. Occlusion of the entire basilar artery is devastating and usually fatal. There is extensive infarction of the midbrain and pons.

The locked-in syndrome is usually produced by basilar thrombosis, although pontine hemorrhage, or central pontine myelinolysis can also produce it. Patients have preserved consciousness but damage to the ventral pons results in inability to respond with movements of the arms and legs. The only preserved movements are vertical eye movements and eye closure. It is easy to overlook the responsiveness and assume the patient is comatose.

Branch occlusion of the basilar artery

Branch occlusions of the basilar artery may produce a variety of syndromes that are more the purview of the neurologist than the generalist. For completeness, some of these are listed in Table 9.2.

Evaluation of stroke

Brain imaging

Almost every patient with stroke requires a brain image. There are occasional patients who are so elderly or physically bulky that scanning is not done. CT is the preferred initial imaging modality for most patients, as CT is able to clearly differentiate hemorrhage from infarction and subarachnoid blood is better visualized on CT than MRI. MRI is often required to delineate the precise nature of the process. Diffusion weighted MR imaging is sensitive to very early infarcts and MR angiography and/or venography may pinpoint the stroke and direct therapy.

Vascular imaging

Ultrasound evaluation of the carotid arteries and heart is performed on most patients with stroke. Carotid duplex ultrasound will show one of five findings:

- normal;
- plaque without significant stenosis;
- high-grade stenosis;
- occlusion; or
- dissection.

Normal findings are often confusing to the patients because the cause of the stroke is not obvious. However, it is explained to patients that there is plaque lining the arteries even in the absence of significant stenosis, and that this and other pathology can be a source for the stroke. It does not require high-grade stenosis to cause a stroke, but high-grade stenosis increases the likelihood for stroke.

Management of carotid stenosis is subject to some individual inter-pretation of the data but a reasonably balanced summary is:

- Stenosis of less than 70% should be treated medically (i.e. antiplatelet drugs).
- Stenosis of more than 70% should be treated surgically if the patient has a life expectancy of more than 5 years, is a good surgi-cal candidate, and has had a stroke or TIA.
- In asymptomatic carotid stenosis story, surgery is considered when the carotid stenosis is 70% or greater, and the patient has a likely life expectancy of more than five years and is a good surgical candidate.

■ Endarterectomy may be performed by an open surgical technique or by interventional methods (i.e. angioplasty with stenting). The risk of operative complications such as cranial nerve palsies is greater with the open technique, but restenosis is more likely after the interventional methods. In a given patient local expertise usually determines which technique is recommended.

Laboratory testing

Routine tests of patients with stroke includes

■ comprehensive metabolic panel;
■ complete blood count;
■ prothrombin and prothrombin–thromboplastin times;
■ ECG;
■ chest x-ray.

Most patients with ischemic stroke should have:

■ Transesophageal echocardiogram
■ Cardiac holter monitor

Additional tests may be required in some patients (e.g. patients with ST changes on ECG may need to rule out myocardial infarction (ROMI) panel and serial ECGs. Young patients or those with other signs suggestive of vasculitis should have a fluorescent antinuclear antibody (FANA) and ESR done, although CNS-angiitis may be associated with normal ESR. Young patients should also undergo a search for a hypercoagulable state, such as antiphospholipid antibiotics, the factor V Leiden or prothrombin gene mutations.

Cerebral angiography is indicated for patients with ultrasound evidence of significant stenosis and in some patients with recurrent stroke despite antiplatelet therapy, or in patients who cannot undergo a less invasive investigation of the blood vessels, such as CT angiography or MR angiography, or if these techniques fail to yield an adequate image for valid interpretation.

Treatment of stroke

Emergency management

The CT scan will differentiate ischemic from hemorrhagic stroke.

Aspirin

All patients with ischemic stroke who are not already on antiplatelets or warfarin (coumadin) should have 150 mg of aspirin administered immediately. While for long-term prevention low-dose aspirin (75–150 mg daily) is just as good as full dose, the initial dose must be sufficient to produce an immediate antiplatelet effect.

Heparin

Patients with progressive deficit are usually started on heparin intravenously, although this is based on limited evidence. Patients with multiple TIAs leading up to stroke are also often treated with heparin.

Tissue plasminogen activator (TPA)

TPA is used intravenously for patients with acute ischemic stroke. Details of the inclusion and exclusion criteria are included in the published prescribing information for TPA, but in brief, the following guidelines must be absolutely met:

- Acute ischemic stroke (less than 3 hours from onset of symptoms);
- Absence of blood, mass or edema on CT;
- No recent surgery;
- No anticoagulants.

Acute stroke means that the patient was last seen to be normal less than 3 hours from the time of administration of the TPA. If a patient went to bed at night and awoke with a deficit, we do not know whether the stroke developed one minute after bedtime or one minute prior to awakening.

Early signs of edema on the CT mean that there has been sufficient damage to the blood–brain barrier that the risk of bleeding with TPA is increased.

In addition, the following features are strongly encouraged:

■ the stroke should not be too severe or too mild;
■ deficit is not substantially improving;
■ no malignancies;
■ not advanced age (i.e. 85 years or more).

If TPA is given, the following regimen is given:

■ Dose of 0.9 mg/kg to a maximum of 90 mg.
■ Bolus is given of 10% of the total dose, with the remainder given over one hour.
■ No anticoagulants are given for 24 hours.
■ Follow-up CT is performed 24 hours later to ensure that there is no bleeding, after which antiplatelet or anticoagulants can be ordered if needed.
■ Patients who receive TPA should be at hospitals where neurosurgical coverage is available, because of the possibility of intracranial hemorrhage.

Blood pressure management

BP is usually elevated in patients with acute stroke. The occlusion of an artery induces elevation in blood pressure to try to force oxygen and nutrients into an area of ischemia. While hypertension is certainly a major risk factor for stroke, acutely lowering the blood pressure may be associated with impaired perfusion pressure, and therefore extension of the infarct. Allow the BP to autoregulate up to about 210/110. If BP exceeds this level and one needs to reduce the BP gently, avoid calcium channel blockers (e.g. nifedipine), and use a short-acting drug such as a beta-blocker such as labetolol.

Prevention of recurrent stroke

Prevention of a first stroke is *primary prevention*. Prevention of a recurrent stroke or TIA is *secondary prevention*.

Prevention of subsequent stroke consists of reduction of blood coagulation and reduction of risk factors. Reduction of coagulation consists of antiplatelet agents and warfarin. Reduction of risk factors consists:

- long term control of blood pressure
- lower cholesterol
- control diabetes
- recognize atrial fibrillation, so that such patients may be treated with long term warfarin.

Antiplatelet agents are effective for patients who are at increased risk of stroke from peripheral vascular disease, cardiac disease, or previous cerebrovascular disease. Use in patients without these events is unproved.

Antiplatelet agents include:

- aspirin
- dipyridamole
- clopidogrel
- ticlopidine.

In addition, there is a popular combination of low-dose aspirin plus high-dose sustained-release dipyridamole (Asasantin Retard).

Aspirin has been shown to reduce the incidence of secondary stroke by 15–19%, depending on the study cited. Aspirin is also used for primary stroke prevention. Also, if the patient cannot afford some of the other agents discussed below, aspirin is certainly better than nothing for stroke prevention.

Dipyridamole is an antiplatelet agent that had largely been ignored after a series of unimpressive studies. However, recent studies have found that high-dose sustained release dipyridamole does indeed reduce the incidence of secondary stroke, and by a proportion which is comparable to the effects of aspirin. The combination of aspirin and sustained release dipyridamole (Asasantin Retard, Aggrenox), reduces the incidence of secondary stroke about 37%.

Clopidogrel is another antiplatelet agent. There is a small risk of thrombocytopenia in patients treated with clopidogrel, although this risk is low enough that routine blood monitoring is not needed.

Thrombocytopenia is much less likely after the patient has been on the drug for a few weeks. The combination of clopidogrel plus aspirin is currently being studied.

Ticlopidine is chemically similar to clopidogrel but has a higher incidence of hematological adverse effects. Because of this, ticlopidine is not widely used. If ticlopidine is used, CBC must be checked every 2 weeks for the first 12 weeks and every 3 months thereafter. The risk of hematological side-effects is much less after the first 12 weeks, although the blood monitoring is still done.

Warfarin (international normalized ratio of 2–3) is used for patients with atrial fibrillation to prevent stroke. In these patients, the risk of stroke is so high that conservative therapy with antiplatelet agents is not warranted unless the risk of using warfarin is excessively high. The main contraindication to the use of warfarin is excessive risk of bleeding. These conditions include some patients with cancers, known GI bleeding, platelet abnormalities, and patients who are non-compliant. These patients have a markedly increased risk of demise with administration of warfarin. Advanced age and ataxia are also relative contraindications.

Transient ischemic attack

TIA is the sudden onset of a neurological deficit that always disappears by 24 hours and usually within 20 minutes. The most important cause by far is carotid artery disease. Transient monocular blindness (amaurosis fugax) is virtually diagnostic of a carotid source. TIAs do occur in the vertebro-basilar territory, but here surgery is not an option and interventional techniques are experimental. TIAs may rarely be cardiac in origin, be caused by blood disorders (e.g. polycythemia) or a primary arteritis and may be the presentation of a 'steal' syndrome.

Rarely, partial seizures, migraine and atypical syncope may be confused with TIAs. The main clue to diagnosis of these is multiple recurrent episodes over time without development of a fixed deficit, especially if refractory to antiplatelet therapy. Neurological consultation is helpful for confirming this diagnosis.

Evaluation of TIA

Recommended evaluation for patients with TIA usually consists of:

- CT head
- carotid ultrasound
- cardiac ultrasound.

The CT is likely to be normal, but should be done to look for tumors or vascular malformations, which can produce symptoms resembling TIA. Young patients should probably have MRI done to look for MS, although very brief symptoms would not be expected to be due to MS. This is more of concern in patients with stroke.

Ultrasounds are done to look for an embolic source, but are less important in patients of advanced age who would not be candidates for anticoagulation or surgery.

Young people should also have additional studies for causes of stroke, including:

- antinuclear antibodies (ANA)
- ESR
- lupus anticoagulant
- protein S and protein C
- anti-cardiolipin antibody
- antithrombin 3
- factor V Leiden mutation
- prothrombin gene mutation.

Angiography is performed when the ultrasound suggests high-grade stenosis or ulcerated plaque and MRI or CTA cannot be done or prove technically inadequate.. If the patient is not a candidate for surgery, due to age or medical condition, there is little point in performing the angiography.

Treatment of TIA

A single TIA can usually be treated with antiplatelet agents while the evaluation proceeds. Aspirin is good enough for primary stroke prevention – when there is a risk of cerebral vascular disease but no definite

TIA or stroke already. If the patient has already had a cerebrovascular event, secondary stroke prevention should involve a combination of antiplatelet agents. Aspirin plus high-dose sustained-release dipyridamole is one of these options.

Heparin is used when there have been multiple TIAs, especially in a short period of time. This results in reduction in the incidence of TIAs and a reduction in the risk of TIA becoming stroke. Unfortunately, the data supporting the efficacy of using heparin in TIA and stroke is weak.

Tissue plasminogen activator (TPA) is not used for patients with TIA. There is no benefit in giving TPA to a patient whose deficit has resolved. In fact, TPA should not be given to patients whose deficit is rapidly improving, for this same reason. TPA is not thought to alter the chance of recurrent stroke or TIA.

Antiplatelet agents are the mainstay of treatment of patients with TIA, and the discussion of these agents is the same as the discussion for stroke, above.

Clopidogrel is used for patients who cannot take aspirin. Although there is little information to support its use other than theoretical, most use low-dose aspirin (81 mg) once daily in addition to the clopidogrel.

Ticlopidine is seldom used, because of the potential for hematological adverse effects.

Warfarin is used predominantly for patients with atrial fibrillation or when antiplatelet agents have failed.

Other than antiplatelet agents and anticoagulants, general risk reduction is key to prevention of recurrent TIA and stroke. Cholesterol-lowering drugs need special mention. The statins are very effective in reducing the risk of secondary stroke. Therefore, the statins are often used even in patients who do not have hypercholesterolemia.

Hemorrhage

Hemorrhage is much less common than infarction, but still represents about 16% of all strokes. The most common hemorrhagic stroke types are:

- subarachnoid hemorrhage
- intraparenchymal hemorrhage
- subdural hematoma
- epidural hematoma.

Suspicion of any of these demands immediate hospital care and specialist consultation.

Subarachnoid hemorrhage (SAH)

SAH is usually due to rupture of a congenital saccular (berry) aneurysm. The onset of symptoms is explosive, patients often describing the sensation as a grenade going off in their head. The onset may be during a period of exertion such as sex or exercise, but can occur at any time. Hypertension and family history predispose to SAH, although some patients have no identified precipitating factors.

Symptoms which should make the generalist worry about SAH are:

- abrupt onset of headache;
- brief loss of consciousness at the time of onset of headache;
- diplopia or other neurological deficit in association with a headache which otherwise seems vascular;
- neck pain associated with the headache;
- duration of the headache for more than 24–48 hours.

Evaluation for possible SAH begins with CT scan. MRI is not as sensitive in detecting subarachnoid blood. CT shows blood in the subarachnoid space in more than 90% of patients with SAH. However, if the CT is negative, then lumbar puncture is needed to rigorously exclude subarachnoid blood.

Intraparenchymal hemorrhage

Intraparenchymal hemorrhage is usually related to untreated hypertension, although vascular malformations can also be implicated. The symptoms depend on the location of the bleeding which is typically in the putamen (50%), thalamus (20%), pons (10%), cerebellum (10%), and lobar (10%). Common symptoms are:

- headache
- nausea and vomiting
- hemiparesis
- decreased level of consciousness
- inability to walk.

CT shows blood in the brain. Because the blood is within the substance of the brain, surgical drainage is avoided unless needed as an immediate life-saving maneuver. The blood is eventually absorbed if the patient survives the acute event.

Subdural hematomas

Subdural hematoma is usually seen after trauma and in the elderly. The bridging veins over the cerebral cortex can rupture producing a slow accumulation of blood which then compresses the hemisphere. There may be a history of trauma, but as often as not the trauma was relatively trivial and often forgotten.

Subdural hematoma presents with signs of increased intracranial pressure:

- headache
- nausea and vomiting
- decreased level of consciousness.

Focal neurological deficits are not as common as with intra-parenchymal hematomas but do occur. Patients often complain of diffuse weakness which may only be recognized as focal upon detailed examination. Seizures may also develop.

Diagnosis of subdural hematoma is usually made by CT. This will determine whether the bleeding is recent, remote, or a combination of the two. Surgical treatment is considered for all but the smallest subdural hematomas.

Epidural hematoma

Epidural hematoma is almost always the consequence of severe head injury. After the injury, the patient may awake (the lucid interval), seemingly unscathed by the injury. Then minutes to hours later he loses consciousness and images reveal the hematoma. There may not be the classic lucid-interval, and the patient may be unconscious from the start.

Occasional patients may have delayed epidural hematoma, with reports of development of bleeding up to 2 weeks after the injury.

When to refer

- abrupt onset of severe headache, suggestive of hemorrhage;
- acute stroke – with acute onset of neurologic deficit;
- multiple TIAs which do not respond to antiplatelet therapy;
- ultrasound evidence of high-grade carotid stenosis or ulcerated plaque.

Pearls

- A completed stroke is often a catastrophe for the patient, with no way of restoring those damaged neurons. Prevention of such disasters is one of our most useful tasks in the practice of general medicine.
- Since 70% of strokes are related to hypertension, the aggressive treatment of hypertension will prevent many such strokes.
- Lipid lowering also contributes to stroke prevention by reducing the progress of atherosclerosis and probably by improving endothelial function.
- Atrial fibrillation demands warfarin unless specifically contraindicated; keep the INR between 2 and 3 to reduce embolic stroke without significantly increasing intracranial bleeding.
- TIA demands urgent evaluation of the carotid arteries. Any suspicion of a TIA as the cause of the patient's symptoms warrants a neurologist and so too do atypical features. The interim medical management is antiplatelet drugs in the form of aspirin 81–325 mg daily.
- Headache with nausea, vomiting, and neurological deficit suggests intracerebral hemorrhage.

chapter 10

Dementia and memory loss

Approach to the patient

IQ testing is possible from about the age of 5. Whatever the outcome of this test, it becomes set for life. Dementia by definition is the loss of intellectual capacity. It is therefore readily distinguishable from mental retardation but need be neither progressive (e.g. brain trauma or ischemia) nor an absolute consequence of ageing.

When a patient presents with a possible dementia, the first question is: Who is complaining? If someone is concerned that their relative might have dementia, they are nearly always right. If the patient himself is concerned he may have dementia he is usually wrong. The adage that you should not worry about Alzheimer's disease because 'if you get it you will never know' is an oversimplification but generally true. Patients with Alzheimer's disease seem generally undisturbed by their bizarre forgetfulness and incongruent behavior. On the other hand the WIGA ('Worried-I've-Got-Alzheimer's') patient is desperately concerned about his failing memory and often resorts to making lists. The WIGA patient is almost always suffering from normal senescent memory change which begins in the 3rd and 4th decades and is, unfortunately, unavoidable.

History and examination

The history pays particular attention to the age of onset (Alzheimer's disease is rare below 60), pre-morbid intellect and personality, speed of onset (Alzheimer's is insidious), and current functional impairment. Also important are current medications, co-existent illness and other symptoms such as bowel and bladder dysfunction. Throughout history taking, the physician is watching for the warning lights, which suggest an alternative diagnosis.

The neurological assessment has four sections:

- *Concentration.* Can the patient maintain a stream of thought or action? For example, simply telling a history to the physician, or on testing, naming animals in order which begin with each letter of the alphabet, or serial sevens (Chapter 1).
- *Language.* The Alzheimer patient, even at a stage of moderate severity, has empty or vacuous speech, with little content. In mild disease, the speech is better but still there are difficulties in expressing oneself and in understanding complex purely verbal commands.
- *Memory.* In casual conversation inquire about events that would normally interest them, for example, sport or politics, depending on their background and checking for memory of recent events. Formal examination of memory includes remembering three objects and a simple story.
- *Visuo-spatial skills.* Ask the patient to copy an abstract diagram or draw the face of a clock including hands to indicate the approximate time.

In the formal neurological assessment, particular attention is given to:

- gait
- coordination of limbs
- visual fields
- funduscopic examination.

Laboratory studies

Patients with suspected pseudodementia require psychological testing rather than laboratory testing, so no laboratory studies are routinely performed. If this evaluation suggests an organic basis, then laboratory studies are ordered. The basic panel of tests for diagnosis of dementia includes:

- chemistries
- complete blood count
- thyroid function tests
- vitamin B12 and folate levels
- serological test for syphilis.

Folate levels are ordered along with the vitamin B12 levels, although isolated folate deficiency as a cause of dementia is not seen. Note that patients may have significant cognitive problems with B12 deficiency without macrocytic anemia or signs of spinal cord and peripheral nerve dysfunction.

A CT should ideally be added to the routine list of tests. However, this need not be done with contrast for most patients, as the main alternative diagnosis, in the absense of focal neurological signs, is normal pressure hydrocephalus.

Differential diagnosis

The diagnosis of specific entities is discussed with the specific conditions, but there are some general guidelines:

- Progressive dementia without other abnormalities on neurological examination is usually Alzheimer's disease.
- Progressive dementia with gait disturbance may be Alzheimer's disease, but normal pressure hydrocephalus (NPH) and Parkinsonism should be considered.
- Dementia with focal or multifocal signs suggests structural CNS lesions such as strokes or masses.

Table 10.1 summarizes the clinical features of some of the important causes of dementia.

Alzheimer's disease

Alzheimer's disease (AD) is the most common cause of dementia, responsible for about half of the cases. If a patient is over the age of 65, has dementia, and an otherwise normal neurological examination, then AD is by far the most likely diagnosis. The other major

Table 10.1 Differential diagnosis of dementia

Disorder	Clinical features	Laboratory findings
Alzheimer's disease	Progressive dementia with intact gait and an otherwise normal neurologic examination	Labs are normal. Scan shows atrophy or is normal
Vascular dementia	Stepwise or gradually progressive dementia with focal or multifocal signs. Vascular risk factors are typically present	Lab is normal or shows risk factors for vascular disease. Scan shows multifocal infarctions which may be large or small vessel
Parkinsonism	Progressive dementia with motor slowing, rigidity, and usually tremor. Postural instability and gait difficulty	Labs are normal. Scan is normal or shows atrophy
Vitamin B12 deficiency	Progressive dementia often with ataxia	Labs show B12 deficiency, although symptoms may develop when the level is in the low-normal range. Scan is normal, but MRI may show white matter changes if the patient has subacute combined degeneration
Pseudodementia of depression	Cognitive difficulty with reduced attention and concentration. Rigorously-tested memory is normal	Labs are normal. Scan is normal
Benign forgetfulness	Memory complaints with totally normal examination. Make sure to reassess in 6 months	Labs and scan are normal
Normal pressure hydrocephalus	Progressive dementia usually with ataxia and urinary incontinence; this is a triad which may not be complete at diagnosis	Labs are normal. Scan shows increased ventricular size, out of proportion to cortical atrophy. Confirmation of diagnosis is by radionuclide cisternography

diagnosis to be considered is pseudodementia. Almost all other causes of dementia are associated with ataxia or other abnormalities on neurological examination.

Diagnosis

The diagnosis of AD is suggested by:

- progressive dementia of at least 6 months duration;
- normal examination other than for mental status including intact gait;
- normal laboratory studies;
- image of the brain is normal or shows atrophy.

There are new tests which can suggest AD, including tau protein, beta peptide, and apolipoprotein-E typing, but these are not definitive, and have no place in routine clinical practice. AD remains a clinical diagnosis.

There are other degenerative dementias including frontotemporal dementia (Pick's disease), dementia with Lewy bodies, cortical-basal degeneration, and progressive supranuclear palsy, but these are less common, and missing these is not fraught with much harm to the patient.

Medical treatment

Treatment of the dementia includes treatment of cognitive deficits and the behavior, as behavioral problems are present in a large proportion of patients.

Treating the cognitive defects

Acetylcholinesterase inhibitors are the mainstay of cognitive treatment. These agents work by increasing the amount of acetylcholine at cholinergic nerve terminals in the brain. In addition, there is some evidence to suggest that there may be a benefit on neuronal degeneration, though this is not proved. Among the benefits of these drugs are:

- improvements in cognitive functioning;
- delay in entry into nursing homes;
- improvement in behavior.

The drugs we use include:

- tacrine (tetrahydroaminoacridine)
- donepezil
- rivastigmine
- galantamine.

The details of these drugs are summarized in Table 10.2.

As these medicines are used, the effect is monitored by assessing cognitive and behavioral performance. Both can be evaluated in part by interview with the caregiver, and this is the only practical way to determine success on activities of daily living. Cognitive performance may be assessed by the mini-mental state examination (MMSE), but studies have not shown this to be an ideal assessment tool, and it is not practical to perform detailed psychometric testing on patients in the clinic. Therefore, the MMSE can be performed, but should not be used as a litmus test to success of the treatment.

Tacrine

Tacrine was the first cholinesterase inhibitor, and is still available. However, it has largely been dropped by most clinicians because of qid dosing, long titration schedule, and required liver monitoring. Dosing is as follows:

- 10 mg qid for 4 weeks
- 20 mg qid for 4 weeks
- 30 mg qid for 4 weeks
- 40 mg qid.

Higher doses are not always used, although most patients do not show benefit unless they are on the upper two doses. Therefore, the dose should be increased if the patient does not respond to the lower doses. Blood monitoring of alanine aminotransferase (ALT) is required every two weeks for the first three months, or for three months after a steady-state dose has been reached. If the ALT increases, the package insert gives precise instructions on modifying the dose. If this drug is used, it is essential to refer to this information and make the appropriate adjustments.

Table 10.2 Drugs used for cognitive treatment of Alzheimer's disease

Generic name	Brand name	Supplied	Dose	Notes
Donepezil	Aricept	Tabs: 5, 10 mg	Start: 5 mg nocte (USA: qhs). After 1 month, inc to 10 mg nocte if needed	Long half-life. Can be given once daily
Rivastigmine	Exelon	Caps: 1.5, 3, 4.5, 6 mg	Start 1.5 mg bid. Increase to next dose at 2 week intervals	Starting dose is not thought to be effective
Galantamine	Reminyl	Tabs: 4, 8, 12 mg	Start: 4 mg bid. Increase to next doses at 4-week intervals if needed	Starting dose is not thought to be effective

Donepezil

Donepezil is an easy-to-use acetyl cholinesterase inhibitor. It is well tolerated with a low incidence of intestinal side-effects. Advantages of donepezil include once-per-day dosing and long half-life.

Dosing is as follows:

- 5 mg at bedtime for 2 weeks, then if needed
- 10 mg at bedtime.

Higher doses have been studied but have not been found to provide improved efficacy. The starting dose of 5 mg at bedtime is effective for many patients, so increasing the dose is not essential unless there is no efficacy.

The half-life of donepezil is long, approximately 70 hours. Therefore, one should stop the medicine for 1 week prior to beginning one of the other cholinesterase inhibitors, to avoid cholinergic crisis.

Rivastigmine

Rivastigmine is a powerful cholinesterase inhibitor that inhibits both acetylcholinesterase and butyrylcholinesterase, which theoretically gives it an advantage over some of the other agents.

Dosing is as follows:

- 1.5 mg bid for 2 weeks, then
- 3 mg bid for 2 weeks, then if needed
- 4.5 mg bid for 2 weeks, then if needed
- 6 mg bid.

This starting dose of 1.5 mg bid is not an effective dose, so patients should have the dose increased unless there are adverse effects. The incidence of intestinal side-effects can be minimized by accelerating the dose slowly, and by administering the drug with food. Sometimes, patients will continue on the drug at a certain dose for up to 4 weeks prior to making an increase. This greatly increases tolerability.

Galantamine

This is the newest of the cholinesterase inhibitors and has a potential advantage over the others in that in addition to its inhibition of acetyl cholinesterase, there is a direct nicotinic effect which may give additional efficacy. However, good head-to-head comparisons between the drugs have not been made, so this is theoretical.

Dosing is as follows:

- 4 mg bid for 4 weeks, then
- 8 mg bid for 4 weeks, then if tolerated
- 12 mg bid.

Response to treatment is assessed 4–8 weeks after arriving at the target dose. The starting dose of 4 mg bid is not usually considered to be an effective dose, so one cannot evaluate efficacy until the higher doses have been given. Even then, improvement may take many weeks.

Behavioral treatment
Behavioral abnormalities include agitation, depression, psychosis, and personality change. The personality changes are difficult for many families to handle, and they are the least amenable to pharmacological treatment.

Agitation
Agitation is best treated non-pharmacologically, if possible. Several suggestions for caregivers are:

- *Distraction.* Identify some basic interests of the patient which can be used to deflect the patient's thoughts from an angry situation. For example, if a patient has a special interest in certain video tapes, playing one of those when tempers are escalating can be helpful.
- *Non-confrontational attitude.* Arguing with a demented patient is seldom helpful, since the patient's disordered thought processes preclude being convinced by logic.
- *Decisions.* People like to make decisions, and the ability to decide between two processes is more attractive than being forced to do one of them. This is true for people of all ages. For example, if it is time for night-time activities, presenting a choice of shower or bath gives an element of self-determination for the patient.

Among the medications which are used are neuroleptics, benzodi-azepines and other anti-anxiety agents, and antidepressants. While these can improve an acute episode of agitation, they take time to work so they may not help an isolated attack. Also, these agents may increase confusion. Antidepressants are most beneficial if used chronically. They are of little value when used as single doses. Some of the commonly used agents are:

- lorazepam
- risperidone
- valproate

Risperidone is often a useful neuroleptic for patients with dementia, especially AD, however, it should not be used for patients with Parkinsonism because of the potential for rigidity and other extrapyra-midal effects. Clozapine, olanzepine and quetiepine are often better when Parkinsonism is a component of the problem.

Valproate is helpful for some patients with intermittent explosive symptoms in association with dementia.

Depression

Depression is a common component of dementia, not only among patients with AD but also in patients with other degenerative demen-tias. Depression is present in patients with or without insight into their disease, indicating that this is not just a reactive mood distur-bance, but rather is an endogenous depression.

Some of the best medicines for depression in the setting of demen-tia are:

- paroxetine
- sertraline
- fluoxetine
- venlafaxine

The first three are SSRIs and the last has multiple neurotransmitter effects. TCAs are typically not used because of the risk of confusion from the anticholinergic effect.

Psychosis

Psychosis is common in patients with dementia, although it is more likely in patients with Lewy body dementia than with AD. Most hallucinations and illusions do not have to be treated, since they are non-threatening. However, if medications are needed, the following can be helpful:

- risperidone
- olanzapine
- quetiepine.

Sleep disturbance

Sleep disturbance includes the spectrum from sleeping all the time to insomnia to nocturnal awakenings.

Excessive sleeping. Stimulants are occasionally used, although they may exacerbate agitation, and are not routinely used by most physicians. Some antidepressants have a stimulating effect. Sertraline has been helpful for many patients.

Insomnia. Insomnia is treated non-medically if possible. Absence of napping and avoidance of stimulating activities and shows before bed can help. Sedative-hypnotics are used sparingly, but can be of benefit. They can occasionally produce a hangover effect, can increase confusion, and there is concern over a potential for increasing gait disorder when patients get up in the middle of the night to use the toilet facilities. Zolpidem and zaleplon may be helpful. TCAs are avoided because of their anticholinergic effects.

Nocturnal awakenings. Nocturnal awakenings can be treated as insomnia, with good sleep hygiene and abstinence from daytime naps. Some AEDs may be helpful for sleep fragmentation, including carbamazepine.

Vascular dementia

Vascular dementia (VaD) has a variety of presentations, and may appear indistinguishable from AD. In fact, patients may have elements of vascular plus degenerative dementia, since even small infarcts may trigger or accelerate the degenerative cascade, which results in degenerative dementias. Therefore, there is some overlap between these entities.

The diagnosis of VaD is suspected when a patient presents with a dementia of step-wise progression or sudden onset. While a single infarct is less likely to produce dementia than multiple infarcts, the onset of the noticed intellectual deterioration may be coincident with a single infarct.

Diagnosis

Diagnosis of VaD is suggested by:

- sudden or step-wise progression of dementia;
- focal or multifocal neurological deficits on examination;
- risk factors for vascular disease;
- imaging signs of multiple infarctions.

Note that patients with extensive small vessel disease or multiple infarctions from atrial fibrillation may have a progressive dementia, where the individual infarctions are not clinically appreciated.

Treatment

No medications have been proved effective for treatment of patients with VaD. Presently, one may:

- reduce risk factors
- reduce recurrent stroke rate by use of antiplatelets and anti-coagulants
- control behavior.

Cholinesterase inhibitors are currently being studied in patients with VaD. However, these have not yet been found to be beneficial.

Normal pressure hydrocephalus

Normal pressure hydrocephalus (NPH) is probably a misnomer. There may be times when intraventricular pressure is high which eventually results in dilatation of the ventricles. The lateral ventricles are mainly affected then the third and fourth ventricles.

Diagnosis

The diagnosis of NPH is suspected when a patient develops dementia and the imaging shows increased ventricular size. Ventricular dilatation is common in degenerative dementias also. However, in degenerative diseases there is cortical atrophy appropriate to the ventricular dilatation. In NPH, the ventricular dilatation is out of proportion to the cortical atrophy.

The typical triad of NPH is dementia, ataxia, and urinary incontinence, but the complete triad is present in a minority of patients, especially early in the course. Laboratory testing is unremarkable but imaging is suggestive. Additional supportive evidence can be gleaned from lumbar puncture with radionuclide cisternography. Removal of CSF (about 30 cc) can produce a clinical improvement, which may be best determined in gait. The radionuclide injected at the time of the LP is followed with serial brain scans over 24 to 48 hours. In patients with NPH, there is reflux of the tracer into the ventricles, rather than the normal migration of tracer rostrally and across the cerebral convexities to the arachnoid granulations. The clinical response to the diagnostic lumber puncture is the most accurate predictor of response to surgical shunting.

Treatment

There are no viable medical treatments for NPH. Surgery can be helpful for some patients with NPH, although there is no guarantee of either beneficial effect or absence of adverse effect. Ventriculo-peritoneal shunting may reduce the ventricular dilatation result in improvement. The gait disorder tends to improve more than the dementia.

Parkinson–dementia complex

Parkinson's disease (PD) is often associated with cognitive disturbance, although not all patients develop dementia. The relative risk of dementia in patients with PD is increased approximately six-fold. The possible reasons for the dementia include:

- Alzheimer's disease coincident with the PD;
- Parkinsonian disorder associated with dementia, such as dementia with Lewy bodies or progressive supranuclear palsy;
- vascular dementia associated with PD as a coincidence.

The markedly increased incidence of dementia in patients with PD compared with age-matched controls suggests that the association is pathological rather than just coincident.

Diagnosis

The diagnosis of PD is discussed in Chapter 11, but the main features are:

- rigidity
- tremor
- loss of postural reflexes
- gait change.

Not all features are present in all patients. The diagnosis is clinical, although some basic tests are required to look for some alternative diagnoses:

- CT to look for NPH or frontal lobe abnormality
- Thyroid function tests

Medical treatment

Treatment of the Parkinsonian features is discussed in Chapter 11 on movement disorders. Treatment of the dementia includes mediations for cognition and behavior.

Treating cognitive deficits

No medications have been approved for use in dementia associated with PD. However, the acetylcholinesterase inhibitors are sometimes helpful. Donepezil and rivastigmine are used in many patients. The magnitude of the cholinergic deficit in some patients with PD is even greater than the cholinergic deficit in patients with AD. The cholinesterase inhibitors used are as presented in Table 10.2.

Behavioral treatment

Patients with PD and dementia are especially susceptible to behavioral abnormalities and psychosis. The dopaminergic agents often make the psychosis worse, especially in patients with advanced disease. Unfortunately, many of the neuroleptics can make parkinsonism worse, so the selection of agents is a little different from the selection for patients with AD. The newer atypical neuroleptics have a lower risk of developing Parkinsonism. Some of the most helpful drugs are:

- olanzepine
- quetiepine
- clozapine.

Clozapine requires blood monitoring, which has reduced the usefulness of this drug.

Depression can be treated by almost any of the modern medications, however, the SSRIs are especially helpful. TCAs are usually avoided because of their strong anticholinergic effect having a deleterious effect on memory.

Other diagnoses to be considered

Subdural hematoma (SDH)

SDH usually presents after an acute head injury, although the onset may be more insidious in the following situations:

- very elderly patients
- patients on warfarin
- patients with a gait disorder.

Older patients have cerebral atrophy which stretches the bridging veins over the cerebral hemispheres. Therefore, even a relatively minor head injury may produce a SDH. Patients on warfarin can ooze blood into the subdural space over weeks, so that the acute onset is not seen. A history of head injury may not be remembered, so patients who have ataxia and a propensity to fall should be considered to be at risk for SDH.

Diagnosis is by brain imaging and treatment is surgical for most patients. With small hemorrhages, surgery may not be necessary.

Brain tumor

Brain tumor is an uncommon cause of dementia. Findings which would suggest tumor include:

- headache
- focal findings on exam with an insidious development
- papilledema.

Olfactory groove meningioma can present with mental status changes without focal findings on examination. Patients usually have a depressed affect and may have other frontal lobe signs including disinhibited behavior. Papilledema may not be present with slowly growing lesions, so scanning is essential to make this diagnosis.

Counseling patients and families

Dealing with the diagnosis

The diagnosis of dementia is devastating to patients and caregivers, but as with any chronic illness, the family can have good quality time during this progression of the condition. Physician assistance during this course is essential. There will be many questions, and the questions will be rephrased and asked again. Eventually, they will deal with the diagnosis as with any chronic illness. A small percentage will develop intractable depression. A larger proportion will become cheerful and life-loving, just requiring some assistance in dealing with the illness.

Information for patients

The diagnosis is established before most information is given to the patient and caregivers. While the family will want to know treatment options and outlook at the earliest visit, the information will be more accurate and the credibility improved when given along with an accurate statement of the diagnosis. The term *Alzheimer's disease* strikes fear into the hearts of many people. Therefore, the term does not always have to be used. *Degenerative dementia* is a term which encompasses Alzheimer's disease as well as a small number of other neurodegenerative diseases, such as frontotemporal dementia. One cannot always distinguish between Alzheimer's and these other disorders so the avoidance of the use of the Alzheimer name is not intellectually dishonest.

Information for caregivers

Patient and caregiver groups often share helpful suggestions for daily living. It can be useful to pass along some of these suggestions to the family in addition to giving them contact information for the local support groups.

A few of the most important suggestions are:

- Don't argue with the patient. The disordered logic processes make rational convincing almost impossible.
- Make bathing a daily routine. Although everyone does not need daily bath (and this is not the norm in many regions of the southern USA), making a daily routine results in eventual less opposition to activities.
- Provide viable options. Allow the patient to make as many decisions as possible, but from a small list of viable options.
- No napping in the day. Well, perhaps a brief rest, but long or repeated naps will interfere with night-time sleep.
- Bed at a rigid time.
- Avoid violent or stimulating television, especially right before bed. This is, of course, less of a problem in the UK than in the USA,

and the availability of programs such as Songs of Praise and Gardener's World provide the ideal visual soporific!

■ Get the patient out of the home daily. Otherwise, the patient may eventually develop a poor tolerance of getting out.

■ Avoid alcohol. Some families, as a sedative and social lubricant, unfortunately use alcohol, but there are potential deleterious effects on the patient including mental status effects and the potential for interference with medications.

■ See an attorney. This is the only time you will find us advocating advocates. There are a number of legal issues which arise and should be dealt with as soon as possible after the diagnosis is made.

■ Patient should not drive. The roads are dangerous enough, what with the drunks, cell-phone talkers, and American tourists all trying to drive on the wrong side of the road.

Role of the GP

The GP is an information resource and rock of stability to the patient and family. Our patients fear uncertainty more than they fear an adverse outcome. How many times have we seen patients deal with a terminal diagnosis better than they did the uncertainty prior to the

Pearls

■ Progressive dementia with an otherwise normal neurological examination is almost always due to Alzheimer's disease.

■ Almost every patient with dementia deserves to have a scan of the brain (CT or MRI).

■ Parkinson's disease has an increased incidence of dementia, and these patients can respond to cholinesterase drugs.

■ Cholinesterase drugs can help more than just cognition, helping behavior and improving performance of activities of daily living.

diagnosis being made? Therefore, even if the physician does not believe that we have anything to offer the patient medically, we are the captains on the ship of life, guiding our patients through the troubled waters, even though we know that iceberg is out there somewhere. The metaphor breaks down since we, as physicians, do not have to go down with the ship. At least, not yet.

When to refer

It is our belief that all patients should have a neurological opinion at some stage. This disease is going to be a long haul and, understandably, the relatives will usually want to hear it 'from the top'. In some areas, imaging can only be obtained through a consultant, and since all patients with AD should have some kind of scan, the neurologist is the ideal expert! Onward referral for neurosurgery where appropriate, or even for psychometric testing, is usually best done via a neurologist.

chapter 11

Movement disorders

Approach to the patient

Most movement disorders are clinical diagnoses. There are no laboratory or imaging studies that will make the diagnosis. They will be
able to demonstrate the cause of a movement disorder in a small
minority of cases.

Classification and diagnosis of movement disorders

Movement disorders can be classified into two general categories:

- too much movement
- too little movement.

Among the patients with too much movement, tremor, myoclonus,
asterixis, chorea, athetosis, dystonia, ballism, akathisia and tic are
examples. Too little movement include bradykinesia, paralysis and
rigidity, topics that are covered elsewhere. Table 11.1 presents some
of the common types of abnormal movements with clinical features
and possible diagnoses. The first task is to classify the movements
into one or more of these categories.

For example, a patient with tremor with rigidity and bradykinesia
likely has Parkinsonism, whereas a patient with tremor without these

Table 11.1 Types of movement disorders

Abnormal movement	Clinical features	Disorders
Tremor	Rhythmic oscillation of the hands or head	Essential tremor, Parkinsonism, enhanced physiologic tremor
Athetosis	Slow twisting, writhing motion	Lesion of the basal ganglia
Chorea	Rapid, jerky movement, often blended into normal movements	Huntington's disease, other basal ganglia lesions
Ballismus	Flinging movements of proximal muscles, may cause injury	Lesion of the subthalamic nucleus, especially stroke
Rigidity	Increased muscle tone with normal or decreased tendon reflexes	Basal ganglia lesions, Parkinsonism, stroke
Spasticity	Increased muscle tone with increased tendon reflexes	Corticospinal tract lesions of the brain, brainstem, or spinal cord. Stroke, trauma, tumor, especially
Dyskinesia	Flapping movements of mainly proximal muscles	Parkinsonism treated with dopaminergic agents, history of neuroleptic use
Dystonia	Increased muscle tone to produce sustained turning or twisting of a limb or head	Drug effect, idiopathic torsion dystonia
Bradykinesia	Slowness of movement	Parkinsonism

features likely has essential tremor. This diagnosis has been made without even knowing the features of the tremor which would differ between these two diagnoses. In that vein, some general guidelines are as follows:

- Resting tremor of the hands is usually Parkinsonism.
- Tremor with movement is usually essential tremor.
- Dystonia without other neurological findings is usually idiopathic torsion dystonia.
- Dyskinesias without signs of Parkinsonism are almost always drug-induced.

What are the common diagnoses?

More than 90% of the patients who present with movement disorder in General Practice will have one of two diagnoses:

- essential tremor
- Parkinsonism.

Patients with Parkinsonism will fall into three general categories:

- Parkinson's disease
- other degenerative disorder with Parkinsonian features
- drug-induced Parkinsonism.

Other degenerative conditions which can present with Parkinsonism include Lewy body dementia, striatonigral degeneration, and multiple system atrophy. However, the GP is not expected to differentiate between these entities, so a limited classification as above is sufficient.

Other diagnoses are much less common, but among these will be:

- tardive dyskinesia
- dystonia.

Dyskinesias will also be seen in patients being treated for Parkinsonism, and when present, the Parkinson's disease diagnosis will be obvious.

Essential tremor

Essential tremor is the most common movement disorder seen in general practice. As a cause for tremor, it is more than ten times more prevalent than Parkinsonism. There is a family history in about 50%, hence the term *familial essential tremor*. The tremor interferes with activities but is seldom disabling, hence the term *benign essential tremor*. However, since it is not always familial and not always benign, we will use the diagnosis *essential tremor*.

Features and diagnosis

Essential tremor is present with the arms outstretched or when manipulating objects. A head tremor (titubation) may be present, although this is not invariable. ET can develop at any age; even children may develop this. In contrast, Parkinson's tremor is usually present in middle aged and elderly patients. While there may be a familial predisposition to Parkinson's disease, essential tremor is more commonly familial.

Examination in ET shows normal motor function except for the tremor with action. Conspicuously absent in a patient with ET are resting tremor of the hands, rigidity, bradykinesia, loss of postural reflexes, cogwheeling, and positive glabellar reflex – all typical signs of Parkinsonism.

Table 11.2 shows important differentiating features between essential tremor and other causes of tremor, including Parkinsonism.

Treatment

Depending on the patient–doctor relationship, essential tremor can be managed by the GP if she is confident in the diagnosis. The most common drugs used for treatment are:

- propranolol
- primidone
- gabapentin
- selected carbonic anhydrase inhibitors.

Table 11.2 Tremor

Features	Essential tremor	Parkinson's tremor
At rest	Absent or only mild head tremor	Pill-rolling tremor of hands
With movement	Tremor superimposed on movement	Tremor lessened, though walking may worsen it
Frequency	5–7 Hz	4–5 Hz
Associated finding	No findings, although tremor may impair fine coordination	Rigidity, bradykinesia, stooped and shuffling gait
Treatment	Propranolol, primidone	Trihexyphenidyl, carbidopa–levodopa

Propranolol and primidone are the most potent. The dose of medication is usually less than that required for other pharmacological events. Efficacy in tremor of propranolol is not based on examination for peripheral beta blockade. For primidone, the doses used are much lower than those required for treatment of epilepsy.

Propranolol
- First-line treatment for most clinicians.
- Low doses are often effective.
- Full beta-blockade is not necessary.
- May be used on an 'as-needed' basis for selected patients.
- Dose of 10–40 mg bid–tid. Higher doses may be tried.

Primidone
- Little used for seizures currently but it is commonly used for essential tremor.
- Doses used are much lower than those used for seizures – 25 mg tid would be a typical dose, increasing to perhaps 250 mg/day if needed.

Gabapentin
- Newly used for patients with essential tremor.
- Dose is typically lower than anti-epilepsy doses. 100 mg tid would be a good starting dose, increasing to a maximum of 2400–3600 mg/day max.
- Lower doses are used in elderly patients and in those with renal insufficiency.

Topiramate
- Recently used for patients with essential tremor.
- Since it is a carbonic anhydrase inhibitor, it increases the risk of urolithiasis, and should not be used in this situation.
- Dose is usually 25 mg daily increasing weekly by 25 mg/day; effective dose for tremor is usually 50–100 mg/day.

Ethanol
Ethanol is frequently an effective treatment for essential tremor for many patients. Unfortunately, this might promote excessive ethanol intake in some individuals.

Parkinsonism

Parkinsonism is one of those diagnoses that is obvious in its advanced form but may be subtle at the time of presentation. In general, labeling a patient as having Parkinson's disease should be reserved for when the diagnosis is certain, since there are many personal and social ramifications of making the diagnosis, and a delay in establishing the diagnosis does not alter the outcome for the patient.

Features and diagnosis
Parkinsonism is a clinical diagnosis. Patients present with any combination of the following:

- tremor
- rigidity
- bradykinesia

- decreased facial expression
- loss of postural reflexes
- gait abnormality
- impaired hand movements.

Tremor is typically 3–5/s pill-rolling tremor which is usually seen in repose when the patient is relaxed. It is often more obvious when the patient is telling the history and not paying attention to the limbs. Movement of the arms damps the tremor but walking often accentuates it.

Rigidity is stiffness of the limbs. This is assessed best by the examiner flexing and extending the elbow when the patient is relaxed. Increased tone is evident with both flexion and extension often with intermittent catches (*cogwheeling*). This rigidity differs from spasticity where there is no cogwheeling, and the stiffness is most prominent in the antigravity muscles and velocity dependent.

Decreased facial expression and bradykinesia produces the masked face which is characteristic of Parkinsonism but can also be seen in patients with depression. Decreased blinking is prominent with Parkinsonism and can be a useful diagnostic feature.

Bradykinesia is slowness of movement and can predate other symptoms by many months.

Gait abnormality with *loss of postural reflexes* gives the patient a tendency to fall which can also predate the other clinical features of Parkinsonism.

Impaired hand movements are typical and best seen with finger tapping and rapid opening and closing of the hands. The magnitude of the finger excursions is impaired and there is poor independent finger movement.

Once the diagnosis of Parkinsonism has been established, the cause should be determined, if possible. The most important question to ask is about a history of drug and toxin exposure. The most important are:

- neuroleptics
- metaclopramide

- carbon monoxide (acute toxicity)
- cyanide (acute toxicity)
- manganese (chronic intoxication)

Tests are seldom revealing in patients with Parkinsonism. If there are prominent unilateral features, then imaging is important to exclude a lesion in the basal ganglia. Hypothyroidism should also be ruled out as a cause for slowness of movement.

A neurologist should be involved early in the course of the illness, not only to support the generalist's diagnosis and exclude the rare causes, but also for moral support. The disease is going to be long and difficult, and may require recurrent consultations.

When deciding on treatment, bear in mind that the negative symptoms of Parkinson's disease (bradykinesia, loss of postural reflexes and the freezing phenomenon) usually cause more distress and therefore warrant more aggressive treatment than the positive symptoms (tremor, rigidity and the flexed posture).

Drug treatment

Drug treatment is presently directed toward symptomatic relief. The improvement in quality-of-life and lessening of disability with the drugs is only from the symptom improvement. No neuroprotective drug currently exists, though candidates are being tested in neurode-generative diseases, epilepsy, stroke and traumatic brain and spinal cord injury.

Selection of individual drugs

The selection of drugs depends on the individual patient situation. To a certain extent, the selection is by trial and error, but some reasoned guidelines can be given. Drugs used for Parkinsonism are summarized in Table 11.3.

Patients who present mainly with tremor may benefit from anti-cholinergic drugs. Dopaminergic agents may be helpful for tremor as well, but are usually used second-line.

Patients who have prominent rigidity and bradykinesia are started on dopaminergic agents. Younger patients are usually prescribed

Table 11.3 Drugs for parkinsonism

Generic name	Brand name	Supplied	Dose	Notes
Levodopa–carbidopa	Sinemet	Tabs: 50–12.5, 100–25, 100–10, 250–25 of each. CR: 100–25, 200–50 mg	Start: 100–25 tid Inc as needed	Dopamine precursor. Note different names for different formulations
Amantadine	Symmetrel	Cap: 100 mg	Start: 100 mg daily. After 1 wk: 100 mg bid. Max: 400 mg/day	Promotes release of dopamine
Ropinerole	Requip	Tabs: 0.25, 1, 2, 5 mg	Start: 0.25 mg tid. Inc weekly. Max: 24 mg/day	Dopamine agonist
Pramipexole	Mirapexin Tolcapone	Tabs: 88, 180, 700 mcg	Start: 88 mcg tid. After 1 wk: 180 mcg tid. Max: 3.3 mg/d total dose	Dopamine agonist
Entacapone	Comtess	Tabs: 200 mg	200 mg with each dose of levadopa. Max: 2000 mg/day	COMT inhibitor. Always given with levodopa
Selegiline	Eldepryl	Tabs: 5 mg. Liq: 10 mg/5 ml	5 mg bid. morning and midday	MAO-B inhibitor
Trihexyphenidyl	Benzhexol/ Broflex Artane	Tabs: 2, 5 mg. Liq: 5 mg/5 ml	Start: 1 mg daily. Inc to 2 mg tid. Max: 15 mg/day	Anticholinergic. Mainly used for tremor

agonists such as ropinerole, pramipexole, pergolide, or bromocriptine. Levodopa is usually used first line for older patients with rigidity and bradykinesia. Levodopa is almost always used with carbidopa, the peripheral dopa-decarboxylase inhibitor, as the combination under the trade name, Sinemet.

As Parkinson's disease progresses, there are frequently fluctuations in the response to levodopa, such that more frequent doses are required. An alternative to frequent dosing is use of a sustained-release version of the levodopa (Sinemet CR). Alternatively, catechol-O-methyl-transferase (COMT) inhibitors can be used to prolong the action of the levo-dopa. The most commonly used of these is entacapone.

Balance is impaired in virtually all patients with Parkinson's disease, but unfortunately, this symptom does not respond well to dopaminergic agents. In fact, if the patient's mobility improves so that they are more ambulatory, they may actually fall more.

Dyskinesias develop in many patients with moderate to advanced Parkinson's disease because of the effects of the dopaminergic agents. This is a sign of dopaminergic over-activity. This responds to lowering of the dose of the dopaminergic agents and may be better with use of a dopamine receptor agonist rather than levodopa, but may also respond to amantadine. Amantadine has some dopaminergic activity on its own, although improvement in rigidity and bradykinesia from amantadine alone is seldom sufficient.

Anticholinergic drugs

The most commonly used anticholinergic drug is trihexyphenidyl (Artane). Starting dose may be as low as 1 mg/day for some patients, although 6–10 mg/day is typical. A usual maintenance dose is 2 mg tid. Doses above 15 mg are unusual for Parkinsonism. Lower doses should be used in patients with advanced age. Some patients may have bladder control complications from use of this class of agents, and they should be warned of this possibility.

Other drugs with anticholinergic effect have benefit, including some in which anticholinergic properties are side-effects such as amitriptyline and diphenhydramine.

Dopaminergic drugs

Dopaminergic drugs include amantadine, dopamine receptor agonists, and levodopa. The specifics on when each of these are used is discussed elsewhere in this chapter.

Note that abrupt withdrawal from dopaminergic agents may be associated with the neuroleptic malignant syndrome. This is especially likely if the patient is on neuroleptics.

Amantadine (Symmetrel)

Mechanism of action: Increases dopa release from the pre-synaptic terminal.

How supplied: 100 mg capsules.

Dose: 100 mg bid may increase to tid if needed.

Indications: Reduced drug-induced dyskinesias. Has some benefit in improving rigidity and bradykinesia.

Adverse effects: Some patients will develop confusion.

Ropinerole (Requip)

Mechanism of action: Dopamine agonist.

How supplied: 0.25, 0.5, 1, 2, 5 mg.

Dose: Increasing dose at weekly intervals as follows:

week 1 = 0.25 mg tid.
week 2 = 0.5 mg tid.
week 3 = 0.75 mg tid.
week 4 = 1.0 mg tid.

Most, but not all, patients will have to escalate the dose to 1 mg tid, and the best response is usually developed by doses of 2 mg tid. or greater.

Indications: For patients with idiopathic Parkinson's disease.

Adverse effects: The most common adverse effects are nausea, dizziness, somnolence, and vomiting. Patients may have symptomatic hypotension. In addition, there have been reports of increased risk of syncope with ropinerole.

Pramipexole (Mirapex)

Mechanism of action: Direct dopamine agonist.

How supplied: 0.125, 0.25, 0.5, 1.0, 1.5 mg tabs.

Dose: Increasing dose at weekly intervals as follows:

week 1 = 0.125 mg tid
week 2 = 0.25 mg tid
week 3 = 0.5 mg tid
week 4 = 0.75 mg tid
week 5 = 1.0 mg tid
week 6 = 1.25 mg tid
week 7 = 1.5 mg tid.

Not all patients need to be escalated to the maximum dose. Most patients require at least 0.75 mg tid to have good benefit.

Indications: For patients with idiopathic Parkinson's disease. Helpful for the rigidity and bradykinesia.

Adverse effects: Can cause confusion in some patients. There are reports of the possibility of symptomatic hypotension. Nausea, sedation, insomnia, and hallucinations were among the most common adverse effects.

Levodopa with carbidopa (Sinemet, Sinemet CR)

Mechanism of action: levodopa is converted to dopamine in the brain. The carbidopa inhibits dopa decarboxylase outside of the brain, thereby reducing intestinal adverse effects of the levodopa.

How supplied: The doses are listed as carbidopa–levodopa as follows: 10–100, 25–100, 25–250, 25–100 CR, 50–200 CR.

Dose: Start at 25–100 tid, and increase as needed. Continuous release

(CR) doses are used if there are fluctuations with the regular dosing. Maximum dose is listed as 2 qid of the 25–250 dose, but few patients will reach this dose.

Indications: For idiopathic Parkinson's disease.

Adverse effects: Nausea is the most common adverse effect. Involuntary movements can develop especially at high doses; these include dyskinesias, dystonic, and choreic movements.

Pergolide (Permax)

Mechanism of action: Dopamine agonist.

How supplied: 0.05, 0.25, 1.0 mg

Dose: 0.05 mg/day × 2 days, then increase by 0.1 to 0.15 mg/day every 3 days for the next 12 days. Then may increase by 0.25 mg/day every 3 days to therapeutic effect. Typical dose will be 1 mg tid.

Indications: For symptomatic improvement of patients with idiopathic Parkinson's disease.

Adverse effects: The most common adverse effects are nausea and other forms of GI distress.

Surgical treatment

Surgery should be considered for patients with advanced Parkinson's disease who have failed medical therapy. Destructive lesions of portions of the internal globus pallidus have been shown to improve various aspects of Parkinsonism. This is most effective for patients with prominent unilateral symptoms, since bilateral surgeries have a higher rate of serious complications. High frequency stimulation of the inner portion of the globus pallidus or sub-thalamic nuclei (deep brain stimulation) produces a functional inhibition of these structures thereby imitating a lesion, but has the advantage of not being destructive. These stimulators can be removed, if ineffective, and can be placed bilaterally.

Stem cell implants have received much attention within the past year, but it will be years before this avenue of treatment is fully developed.

Bottom lines

- Parkinson's disease is a progressive neurodegenerative illness. Treatment improves the symptoms but there is no way to prevent progression. This fact is lost on many patients, whose expectations are unrealistic, expecting that the treatments will prevent progression of the disease.
- Activity is important for preservation of function in Parkinson's disease. Make sure that the patient continues to walk and get out as much as possible.
- There is no single definitive test for Parkinson's disease. This is a clinical diagnosis.
- The patient and his family will need lots of support and help with day-to-day problems. The Parkinson's Society and self-help groups may prove helpful for certain patients.

Other movement disorders

Parkinson's disease and essential tremor are the most common movement disorders. Perhaps next in line is spasticity. While this is not typically classified as a movement disorder, it is a condition of excessive muscle contraction and can be confused with extrapyramidal rigidity, so it will be discussed below. Table 11.4 presents differentiating features between Parkinsonian rigidity and spasticity.

Rigidity implies increased muscle tone and may be due to extrapyramidal or pyramidal dysfunction. In general, rigidity of extrapyramidal origin is bilateral, although often asymmetric, associated with cogwheeling, and may be associated with resting tremor. Reflexes are normal or reduced because of the increased tone.

In contrast, pyramidal dysfunction is associated with increased tone of antigravity muscles with increased reflexes and upgoing plantar responses (Babinski sign).

Bradykinesia is slowness of movement. While it co-exists with rigidity in patients with Parkinson's disease, they have different characters. Bradykinesia is also associated with difficulty initiating

Table 11.4 Differentiation between rigidity of Parkinsonism and spasticity

Feature	Parkinsonism	Spasticity
Lesion	Basal ganglia	Corticospinal tract, anywhere between the cerebral cortex and spinal cord
Muscle tone	Increased in all muscles	Increased especially in antigravity muscles
Cogwheeling	Present	Absent
Tremor	Usually present at rest	Usually absent; may be some action tremor
Reflexes	Normal or decreased by the increased tone	Increased, and may have a clonic component to the reflex
Plantar response	Flexor	Extensor

movements, such as the patient who stands and takes a long time to begin walking.

Too much movement can be due to many different kinds of movement including tremor, akathisia, dystonia, athetosis, chorea, ballismus, dyskinesia, and tics. While conditions such as seizures technically is too much movement, this is not considered here.

The key to diagnosis is correct classification of the movement disorder.

Spasticity

Spasticity is due to damage to corticospinal tract axons. The lesion can be anywhere from the cerebral cortex to the spinal cord. Muscles are stiff because of altered control over spinal reflex pathways. In general, antigravity muscles are overactive. Reflexes are hyperactive and may be clonic – a rhythmic movement is elicited by the hammer tap. Babinski sign is typical although not invariable.

Spasticity is differentiated from rigidity of Parkinsonism by:

- absence of cogwheeling
- reflex abnormalities
- clonus.

Spasticity is differentiated from dystonia by the prominent extensor posturing and abnormal reflexes including Babinski signs.

Treatment with spasticity begins with stretching of affected limbs several times per day. Without this, the muscles can develop permanent contractures. If the patient and family cannot do this, physical therapy may be needed. Medications for spasticity include the following:

- baclofen
- tizanidine
- diazepam
- botulinum toxin
- dantrolene.

There are some other agents which are used and most of these are muscle relaxants. Botulinum toxin is only given by injection into the muscle at the region of the motor endplate and is performed only by neurologists and other trained specialists. This is indicated only for people who need treatment mainly in only one or a few muscles. Details of use of these medications are presented in Table 11.5.

Dystonias

Dystonias are sustained, often twisting, contractions resulting in abnormal body position, as in torticollis. Blepharospasm and writer's cramps are other common examples. Advances in treatment (e.g. botulinum toxin injection), mean that the patient, if distressed by his symptoms, is best referred even if there are no other abnormalities. Athetosis, a slow writhing movement, is a 'moving dystonia' which affects distal muscles, but as such is not really different from dystonia.

Diagnosis

Diagnosis of dystonia based on the history and clinical examination. In general, most juvenile dystonias are idiopathic and most of those inherited.

Imaging of the brain is indicated especially for consistently focal dystonias. Tumors, multiple sclerosis, and other subcortical lesions are unusual, but those diagnoses would change the management. A wide variety of metabolic disorders can be sought, but most of these have other clinical findings which help narrow the diagnostic tests required. Referral is recommended for these dystonias.

Treatment

The most effective treatment for patients with focal dystonias is botulinum toxin injection. These injections are easy, but should all be given by specialists trained and experienced in administration. The injections are given every three months, with the details of administration varying depending on response. Rarely, patients may develop weakness in injected muscles, and there is no treatment for this other than waiting for the toxin to dissipate.

Medical treatment for dystonia consists mainly of anticholinergic agents. Trihexyphenidyl may be slightly effective in doses of

Table 11.5 Drugs for spasticity

Generic name	Brand name	Supplied	Dose	Notes
Baclofen	Lioresal	Tab: 10 mg. Liq: 5 mg/ml	Start: 5 mg tid. Max: 100 mg/day	Available for IV or intrathecal use
Tizanidine	Zanaflex	Tab: 2, 4 mg	Start 2 mg daily. Increase to tid. Max: 36 mg/day	Monthly liver enzymes
Diazepam	Valium	Tab: 2, 5 mg	Start 2 mg tid. Inc as needed. Max: 60 mg/day	Available for IV or IM administration
Dantrolene	Dantrium	Cap: 25, 100 mg	Start: 25 mg daily. Inc to tid. Max: 100 mg qid	
Botulinum toxin	Botox	Vial: 100 units	Injection into muscle q3mo, as needed	Specialist administration only

6–40 mg/day. Adults are usually started on 2 mg tid, and the doses gradually increased. Adverse effects are dose limiting, with many elderly patients unable to tolerate even moderate doses.

Some children with dystonia will respond to dopa ('dopa-responsive dystonia'). It is difficult to diagnosis without trying the medications, so a therapeutic trial is warranted for most children with otherwise idiopathic dystonia.

Localized muscle contractions

Fibrillation
This is the contraction of a single muscle fiber and can only be detected by an electromyographic (EMG) study. Fibrillation potentials are a sign of fluctuation in muscle fiber membrane potential. These potentials are always pathologic and indicate either denervation of muscle, often due to neuropathy.

Fasciculation
Fasciculations are detectable clinically and represents the discharge of anterior horn cells. If not associated with weakness or atrophy, they are likely to be physiological. A simple muscle cramp is a series of fasciculations. Fasciculation can sometimes be elicited by tapping gently with a patellar hammer and may indicate electrolyte disturbances – especially low magnesium. The fasciculation/cramp phenomenon may sometimes be treated with sodium channel blockers (e.g. quinine), antiepileptic drugs (e.g. phenytoin) or magnesium.

Myoclonus and asterixis
The sudden discharge of anterior horn cells producing a sharp movement is called myoclonus and if unassociated with other symptoms or signs is often physiological (e.g. sleep jerks and hiccup). It's counterpart, asterixis, in which the anterior horn cells briefly cease electrical activity, is often seen with myoclonus.

The myoclonus/asterixis phenomenon should raise the spectre of metabolic encephalopathy (e.g. hepatic failure, pulmonary disease, opiate intoxication, uremis). When asymmetric the possibility of a focal brain disease (e.g. stroke) or neurodegenerative condition (e.g. prion disease) should be considered.

Diagnosis
Diagnosis is clinical, with typical appearance of the movement. EEG is frequently obtained to look for seizure activity. A brain image is usually obtained to search for focal structural abnormalities. Laboratory tests should screen for especially hepatic, renal, and electrolyte abnormalities.

Treatment
Treatment consists of resolution of the offending metabolic disturbance, if present. Symptomatic improvement can be seen with valproate or benzodiazepines, although the former may promote a different type of tremor in some patients.

Chorea
Chorea is rapid, purposeless movements involving any part of the body. It may be seen as part of Huntington's disease, systemic lupus erythematosus, benign as in chorea gravidarum. Interestingly, oral contraceptives can bring on the latter. 'Ballism' is a variety of chorea in which violent flinging movements of the limb occur. This bespeaks a lesion of a subthalamic nucleus.

Diagnosis
Diagnosis of chorea is clinical. Patients cannot hide the clinical appearance of the chorea and will be symptomatic during evaluation. Diagnostic tests are performed to look for reversible causes of the chorea, including brain imaging for focal lesions. Genetic testing may be warranted if the differential diagnosis includes Huntington's disease, although this is a controversial area.

Most patients with chorea should be referred for neurological evaluation and initiation of treatment.

Treatment

Management of chorea is usually symptomatic, since a reversible cause is seldom identified. Anti-dopaminergic agents are most effective including neuroleptics (e.g. haloperidol) and dopamine depletors (e.g. tetrabenazine, reserpine). Stereotactic thalamotomy is considered in disabling refractory cases, but is not commonly performed.

Akathisia

A feeling of wanting to move; this may be a neuroleptic side-effect (tardive akathisia), but Ekbom's syndrome (restless legs) is very common and mandates a blood test for iron deficiency. Restless leg is readily treated with a dopamine agonist (e.g. pramipexole), or a benzodiazepine (e.g. clonazepam).

Diagnosis

The diagnosis of akathisia is clinical. All patients should be asked about a history of neuroleptic use. Other agents, which may promote akathisia, include droperidol, prochlorperazine, lithium, and metaclopramide.

Treatment

Management of akathisia begins with discontinuation of the offending agent(s). Fortunately there are a variety of alternatives to neuroleptics. Benzodiazepines and valproate may be effective in the treatment of akathisia.

Tics

Tics or complex movements (habit spasms) associated with a feeling of compulsion to perform them. Sometimes expletives (coprolalia) may be part of the disorder, which is also known as the Gilles de la Tourette syndrome

Diagnosis

Diagnosis of tics is clinical. There is no blood test or image that can rule-in tics. With a good history and observation of the movements, lab tests are usually not needed. Occasionally EEG is done to look for the possibility of seizure activity, but while seizures have many different potential forms, they rarely look like motor tics.

To differentiate motor tics from seizures:

Tics:

- occur when awake;
- increased by stress and can be suppressed voluntarily;
- change in character and distribution over time.

Seizures:

- occur while awake and asleep;
- no consistent effect of stress, and patients cannot suppress them voluntarily;
- tend to be stereotyped in a single patient, although the appearance may differ markedly between patients.

Note that EEG is not required for differentiation in this scheme.

Treatment

Treatment of motor tics is often not needed. The tics tend to be most prominent in teen years then abate with increasing age. Unfortunately, cruel children may make young patients require therapy in order to suppress the tics. One should encourage patients to deal with the tics without medication, but this is not always realistic.

Among the medications used for tics are:

- haloperidol
- pimozide
- risperidone
- clonidine
- clonazepam.

The first three are neuroleptics, and as such are the most effective but do have some small risk of extrapyramidal side-effects. The latter two are our first choices for many patients.

Clonidine

The dose is 0.05–0.1 mg daily to start, progressing to bid maximum dose is 0.3 mg bid, although it is almost never necessary to go to high doses.

Clonidine is beneficial not only for the motor tics, but also may help the hyperactivity, which can coexist with tics.

Clonazepam

The dose is 0.5 mg at bedtime, gradually increasing to a maximum of 6 mg/day in divided doses.

Clonazepam improves the motor tics in many patients and may have some effect on hyperactivity, but it is unacceptably sedating for many patients.

Neuroleptics

The neuroleptics are effective in reducing the tics, and pimozide is the most commonly used. Haloperidol probably has a higher risk for extrapyramidal adverse effects. Risperidol may also be useful but good evidence is lacking.

Stimulants

Stimulants are not used for the motor tics, but rather for the hyperactivity which frequently accompanies tics. Unfortunately, the stimulants often exacerbate the tics. Methylphenidate the most commonly used agent.

Pearls

- Tremor with action and posture is often essential tremor.
- Tremor in repose is usually Parkinsonism.
- Parkinson disease and drug-induced Parkinsonism cannot be differentiated by clinical presentation.

When to refer

- Diagnosis is in doubt.
- The patient fails to respond to treatment.
- Failing doctor–patient relationships.

chapter 12

Case studies

Diabetic neuropathy

Presentation

Ms. Jones is a 57-year-old woman who complained of burning feet. She has had numb toes for 6 months, although she had attributed it to age. Over the past 2 months she has had worsening pain on the bottom of the feet which is now spreading to the top of the feet. Her hands are not apparently affected. No other precipitating factors were identified. Specific negatives were:

- family history of any neuropathic symptoms;
- polyuria and polydipsia;
- occcupational or recreational exposure to heavy metals;
- symptoms of neoplasms;
- significant weight gain or loss;
- unusual dietary/nutritional habits;
- back pain.

Examination shows reduced pin-prick sensation on the top and bottom of the feet with impaired sharp-dull discrimination. Vibration sensation is also decreased. Proprioception is normal. There is subtle reduction in pin-prick sensation on the palms of the hands which is a surprise to the patient. Motor strength and the remainder of the examination is normal. Tendon reflexes are absent at the Achilles tendon and reduced at the patella, but otherwise normal.

Diagnosis

Peripheral neuropathy is suspected on the basis of the distal sensory symptoms and reduction in distal reflexes. The diagnosis is confirmed by EMG, with the report indicating 'Peripheral neuropathy with predominantly axonal involvement'. Laboratory studies to look for reversible causes include:

- chemistries
- complete blood count
- B12 and folate levels
- serological test for syphilis
- thyroid function tests
- serum immunoelectrophoresis

All of the studies are normal except for a glucose of 10.3 mon/L (186 mg/dl) on the fasting chemistries. Follow-up on this with HgBA1C and glucose tolerance test confirms mild diabetes mellitus.

The diagnosis is diabetic peripheral neuropathy.

Management

Management of the diabetes is provided along with counseling on diet and medications when needed. The patient is instructed in foot care to avoid damage to the feet because of the decreased sensation.

The pain is treated with low-dose amitriptyline, starting at 10 mg at bedtime. The dose is increased to 50 mg at bedtime over three weeks, and the patient has good relief of the pain.

Clinical course

Over the ensuing two years, the neuropathy gradually becomes worse, with an increase in the pain necessitating an increase in the dose of amitriptyline. Eventually, a dose of propoxyphene at bedtime has to be added so that she can sleep at night. The escalating doses of amitriptyline cause problems with concentration so the dose is cut back sharply and gabapentin is added beginning at 100 mg tid. This dose is increased until there is again good control on 1200–1800 mg/day. If the patient fails this treatment, other options for management would include carbamazepine or oxcarbazepine.

Discussion

The patient presented with signs of a sensory neuropathy. Few other conditions would produce these symptoms. Diabetes is the most common cause for neuropathy in the developed world, and needs to be sought. Familial neuropathy is another important potential cause, so this is pursued with a careful family history. The immunoelectrophoresis is performed to look for paraprotein which can produce neuropathy. The only study not performed on this patient which might have been justified clinically would be a 24-hour urine test for heavy metals. This is most important in patients who have a risk of exposure in the home or on the job.

The EMG was confirmatory of neuropathy in this patient but may be negative, since small-fiber neuropathy can result in a perfectly normal routine EMG. Therefore, this becomes a clinical diagnosis. With this in mind, EMG is not absolutely essential when there is no motor loss.

The selection of amitriptyline for the burning pain is fine, and gabapentin would have been an alternative. Doses which are required for pain are generally less than the doses required for depression and seizures, respectively. The dose of amitriptyline had to be reduced because of adverse effects, a common occurrence. Addition of gabapentin to the amitriptyline is a good choice since they have differing mechanisms of action. Subsequent discontinuation of the amitriptyline is reasonable though many patients require both drugs.

Epilepsy

Presentation

A 23-year-old woman presents with a single generalized tonic-clonic seizure while sleeping. The duration was only about 10 minutes, and her husband said that she was confused for about one hour afterwards. By the time she awoke in the morning she was completely normal.

No precipitating factors were identified including specific questions about:

- alcohol intake
- illicit drug use
- family history
- history of head injury
- fever, headache, or other signs of brain infection prior to the seizure.

Diagnosis

CT scan of the head was normal. EEG was normal. Routine chemistries and complete blood count were normal. Urine drug screen and blood alcohol levels were also normal.

The diagnosis of a single unprovoked generalized tonic-clonic seizure was made.

Management

The patient was counseled that there was a chance of a recurrent seizure, and that the probability was between 30 and 70%. Therefore, the occurrence of a second seizure was not certain. The physician and patient together decided to not treat the seizure, reserving treatment until a second seizure should occur. Typical seizure precautions were given, including not driving until the physician advised otherwise.

Clinical course

The patient did well until 2 months later when she had a second generalized tonic-clonic seizure. This time the seizure occurred when she was at the market. By the time she was examined, she was normal except for some soreness of the muscles and injury to the tongue.

The patient was placed on carbamazepine 100 mg bid which after one week were increased to 100 mg tid. Levels were checked and eventually became stable and therapeutic on 200 mg tid. She had no further seizures. The plan was to keep her on carbamazepine for at least two years.

Two months later, the patient became pregnant, and by the time of the visit, she was half-way through the first trimester. Prenatal vitamins including folate supplementation were begun. The level of carbamazepine was checked and the dose adjusted. The patient was advised of the effect of epilepsy and anticonvulsants on the fetus.

The carbamazepine level was monitored during the remainder of pregnancy, and the dose had to be increased twice. During the last two months of pregnancy, the dose was not increased despite the level decreasing to the lower limit of the therapeutic range.

Following delivery, the dose of the carbamazepine was reduced to the pre-pregnancy amount, and the blood checked during the first few postpartum weeks to ensure therapeutic levels. The baby was fine.

Discussion

The decision to withhold treatment when a patient has a single unprovoked seizure, a normal examination, and normal diagnostic studies has to be individualized. It is reasonable to avoid AEDs unless indicated by an abnormality on these studies or a subsequent seizure. Occasional patients who demand maximal protection against recurrent seizures will be placed on AEDs after a single seizure, but this should be discouraged.

The pregnancy is problematic, as there are a number of factors to consider. First, this patient was not on an oral contraceptive, but if she had been, the institution of carbamazepine could have decreased the effectiveness several-fold, because of induction of metabolism. Therefore, women of childbearing potential who have epilepsy should always be advised that:

- AEDs reduce the effectiveness of oral contraceptives, usually requiring an increased potency formulation.
- AEDs increase the incidence of some birth defects, and this increase can be reduced, though not eliminated by folate

supplementation, but the folate supplementation must precede the pregnancy. It is too late after the pregnancy is diagnosed.

- Epilepsy increases the risk of obstetric complications including some birth defects, independent of the effects of the AEDs.
- Despite these concerns, most pregnancies in epileptics are uneventful and result in a normal child.

The dose of carbamazepine increased throughout the pregnancy, but in the last two months, the mother's metabolism changes so that she makes high amounts of a metabolite which have significant side-effects. Therefore, the carbamazepine dose should not be increased during this period unless necessary, and should be kept at the lowest effective dose.

Amyotrophic lateral sclerosis

Presentation

A 56-year-old man presented with diffuse weakness which had been progressive for about five months. He noted the weakness first in his hands, with poor strength and coordination for fine activities. No precipitating factors were identified. In addition, he complained of muscle cramps in the arms and the legs.

Further questioning finds that he also has some numbness of the palms which has been present off-and-on for years, and is worse with driving and can occasionally wake him from sleep. There are no bowel or bladder control problems.

Exam shows weakness and wasting of the hands, with both median and ulnar innervated muscles affected. There is subjective decrease in sharp sensation on the palms of the hands bilaterally. Reflexes are increased, there is clonus at the ankles, and bilateral Babinski signs are present. Careful observation reveals fasciculations in the biceps, quadriceps, and calf muscles.

The presence of both upper and lower motorneuron signs is worrisome for motorneuron disease, particularly amyotrophic lateral sclerosis. The numbness would be unrelated, probably due to carpal tunnel syndrome. The differential diagnosis would be peripheral neuropathy with both motor and sensory involvement, though this would not explain the corticospinal tract signs.

Diagnosis

EMG is ordered which shows denervation in all extremities plus bilateral carpal tunnel syndrome. Other sensory nerves are not affected. The electromyographer is concerned about motorneuron disease plus superimposed carpal tunnel syndrome.

X-rays of the neck are done to look for severe spinal degenerative or destructive processes, in case this might account for the corticospinal tract signs. These are unremarkable. Vitamin B12 level and serum lead levels are unremarkable.

The diagnoses of ALS and carpal tunnel syndrome are made.

Management

Riluzole is begun to attempt to slow the progression of the disease. The patient is advised of the side-effects and blood monitoring which is required. In addition, a thoughtful discussion of ALS is made with the patient. For the muscle cramps, phenytoin is prescribed. The patient is also counseled about the progression of the disease.

Clinical course

The patient has relief of the cramps with the phenytoin. The patient gradually declines during the subsequent three years, eventually progressing to the point of being unable to ambulate. Speech and swallowing deteriorate. The patient expires during a bout with aspiration pneumonia.

Discussion

Earlier in this book we discuss the 'heartsink' patient where the physician does not want to face the patient. This is often the case not only for patients with functional disease but also with horrible incurable diseases. The diagnosis of ALS was expected when the patient presented with weakness and hyperactive reflexes with Babinski signs. Most other neuromuscular causes of weakness produce decreased reflexes rather than increased reflexes. The sensory findings represented an inconsistency, but the fact that they seemed to be explained by carpal tunnel syndrome and predated the motor symptoms by such a long time indicated that the motor and sensory symptoms were likely unrelated.

The only test which might have been performed during the initial diagnostic evaluation was an image of the cervical spine. As the patient did not have brainstem dysfunction at the time of presentation, the possibility of a lesion in the cervical spinal cord has to be considered. X-ray would not necessarily rule this out. The EMG findings of denervation in muscles would argue against myelopathy, though.

Riluzole is the only medication which has been proven to slow the progression of ALS. The effect is mild, however, so there is not a life-or-death difference if the patient cannot take it. Other medications such as gabapentin have been studied, but they have no proved benefit.

Counseling patients with ALS is difficult and requires tact and sympathy. For the vast majority of patients this is a death sentence which will not allow them to live more than a few years. However, all hope should not be taken from the patient. Everyone who treats large numbers of patients have had patients who carry the diagnosis of ALS and yet live many years. The reason is that there are other conditions of motorneuron degeneration which can give the same presentation and laboratory findings without the rapid progression of ALS.

Parkinson's disease

Presentation

A 71-year-old man presented with difficulty walking which he had had for 6 months, gradually getting worse. No precipitating factors were identified. No numbness or weakness was noted, and he did better when he had been walking for a few minutes.

His current medications are propranolol for blood pressure control and combination amitriptyline plus perphenazine for sleep.

The exam shows stiffness of all extremities and some cogwheeling with movement at the elbow. Finger tapping and other aspects of fine finger movements are clearly impaired. Gait shows shuffling gait, stooped posture and decreased arm swing. Positive glabellar reflex. No tremor is seen.

Diagnosis

The provisional diagnosis of Parkinsonism has been made. The cause is not clear, but could be related to the perphenazine. Lab studies include thyroid function tests and B12 levels and are normal. CT of the head is done and is normal.

The working diagnosis is Parkinsonism which can be drug related or due to Parkinson's disease.

Management

The perphenazine is stopped, and the patient counseled that this might improve symptoms within the next two months, but this was not certain. The decision was made to hold-off on starting any dopaminergic drugs until this issue had been settled. Activity was encouraged.

Clinical course

Two months later, the patient returns and is markedly improved. It is obvious from just watching the patient enter the room that gait is better. There is still a little increase in tone, but this is not definitely abnormal. Arm swing during gait is still reduced and posture is still stooped, but these symptoms are improved as well.

The presumptive diagnosis of drug-induced Parkinsonism is made, and the patient reassured that continued improvement could be anticipated. Follow-up appointment is scheduled for 6 months.

One year later the patient returns, this time with Parkinsonian features even more prominent than on the initial visit. Posture is stooped with shuffling gait and times when his feet seem glued to the floor. There is a small amount of resting tremor which is less with arm action and greater with gait. Stiffness and cogwheeling in the arms are even more prominent.

The diagnosis of Parkinson's disease is made and the patient begun on carbidopa–levodopa combination at 25:100 tid. This results in some improvement. Over the ensuing two years, the dose has to be increased, and eventually the patient develops rhythmic tremor which is high amplitude and more prominent proximally than distally. The diagnosis of drug-induced dyskinesia is made and the dose of carbidopa–levodopa decreased. Amantadine 100 mg bid is added and he does well for a while. Eventually, the stiffness and bradykinesia gets worse, and he is placed on ropinirole. He receives good response on a dose of 1 mg tid, and the carbidopa–levodopa is decreased.

Discussion

Parkinsonism is one of those conditions which an experienced clinician can diagnose immediately upon meeting the patient, even before taking a comprehensive history and performing an examination. The posture, masked face, and tremors give away the diagnosis. The most common cause of Parkinsonism is Parkinson's disease, an idiopathic degenerative disorder. However, drug-induced parkinsonism is also common, with the main offending agents being neuroleptics and metaclopramide. In general, drug-induced Parkinsonism is less likely to be associated with tremor than Parkinson's disease. However, there is no way to definitively differentiate idiopathic from drug-induced Parkinsonism. Even laboratory tests and images are not diagnostic. Therefore, offending agents should be discontinued. Patients should be advised that improvement after discontinuation of the drug may not begin for weeks, and can take months.

The clinical course documented here is quite typical, with the patient showing initial improvement but then worsening again. This means that the patient was developing the incipient neuronal degeneration of Parkinson's disease when he developed drug-induced

Parkinsonism. Although there was an improvement when the exacerbating drug was discontinued, the degeneration eventually caught up with him and he progressed. The neuroleptic did not have an effect in initiating or accelerating the degeneration.

Patients with Parkinson's disease are treated as discussed in Chapter 8, but in brief:

- young patients are treated with dopamine receptor agonists;
- older patients are treated with levodopa-carbidopa;
- tremor is treated with anticholinergic agents.

The development of dyskinesias is common, and more prominent later in the disease course. High doses of dopaminergic agents produce the tremor. Some ways to minimize the dyskinesia are:

- add amantadine;
- reduce the levodopa to the lowest amounts which maintain function;
- use a dopaminergic agonist with less or no levodopa.

Alzheimer's disease

Presentation

A 75-year-old women is brought by her daughters for evaluation of memory loss. The memory loss has been present for about one year, with a gradual reduction in her activities. She can no longer keep track of her own checkbook and has left food on the stove causing some minor fires in the house. She has had a couple of minor motor vehicle accidents, but none that resulted in serious injury to herself or others.

Exam finds marked deficit in short-term memory with lesser deficit in long-term memory. Speech is halting with incomplete sentences and phrases which seem in poor context and relatively devoid of content. There are no other abnormalities on examination.

The provisional diagnosis of Alzheimer's disease is made.

Diagnosis

A CT of the brain shows diffuse atrophy but is otherwise normal. Thyroid function tests and vitamin B12 levels are also normal. These negative data are supportive of the diagnosis of degenerative dementia and in the absence of other findings on examination, the diagnosis of Alzheimer's disease is made.

Management

The patient and family are counseled on self-care issues, recommendation of seeking legal consultation for finances and end-of-life decisions, and considering alternative residential arrangements so that she is not a danger to herself around the house. Similarly, the patient is advised not to drive because of the risk to herself and others on the road.

The patient are begun on donepezil after neurological consultation and there is some improvement on 5 mg at bedtime. After four weeks the dose is increased to 10 mg at bedtime with some further improvement.

Clinical course

The patient does well for several months, with improvement in function, but eventually declines to the point that she is becoming agitated and hard to manage at home. She has moved in with one of her daughters, and is wearing out her welcome by her behavior. She is started on risperidone 1 mg at bedtime for the agitation with some relief. The plan is to increase this if needed for further control.

The patient eventually progresses to the point of total dependency and has to be placed in a nursing home. Upon entry the donepezil is discontinued. The risperidone has to be increased for a time but then the patient becomes apathetic and less mobile so that the neuroleptic does not have to be continually given.

Discussion

Dementia with a non-focal examination is almost always Alzheimer's disease. Most other causes of dementia are associated with other findings. The other main differential diagnosis would be pseudodementia of depression, but this does not appear to be present in this patient.

Acetylcholinesterase inhibitors such as donepezil slightly improve cognition and performing activities of daily living, such as self-care functions. They have been proven to keep patients out of nursing homes for almost two years, in comparison with non-treatment.

Neuroleptics should be avoided, but occasionally have to be used for patients with paranoia and agitation with dementia. If the patient has Alzheimer's disease or some other condition where there are no Parkinsonian features, then treatment with risperidone is usually considered first. If the patient has Parkinsonian features, then treatment with olanzapine or quetiapine is preferable.

At the point of entry into a nursing home, donepezil and other cholinesterase inhibitors should be discontinued. At this point the patient has ceased to benefit from the drugs.

Headache

Presentation

A 26-year-old woman presents with headaches. The headaches are in the frontal region behind the right eye. They are never on the left. The headaches occur about four times per month and usually occur around the time of menses. She has pounding pain with nausea and vomiting, photophobia and phonophobia. In between headaches, she feels fine and has no complaints.

Neurological and general medical examinations are normal. The clinical diagnosis of migraine is made.

Diagnosis

With episodic headaches of a vascular character and a normal examination, no tests are performed. The clinical diagnosis of migraine headache is felt secure.

Management

The headaches respond to sumatriptan tablets but the patient complains that even having four headaches per month interferes with her job. She is given verapamil as a sustained-release formulation and the number of headaches is reduced by 50%.

Clinical course

She does well for about eight months with a few headaches. However, one week she has a constant headache with neck pain. The pain is not involving the whole head and is associated with nausea and vomiting. Repeated trips to the doctor for relief have been fruitless. In the clinic she has a mild fever and a WBC of 2.1. CT of the head is done to look for mass lesion or blood and is normal. LP is performed which shows a lymphocytic pleocytosis suggestive of fungal meningitis. HIV testing is positive and vigorous antifungal treatment is begun.

Discussion

Migraine is a clinical diagnosis. With a normal examination, diagnostic tests are seldom needed. If she improves then no work-up is done. If she fails to improve, imaging and lab or neurological consultation is warranted.

Treatment with prophylactic medication is usually considered when a patient has four or more headaches per month. The acute attacks may be treated also. If the patient has less frequent attacks, abortive therapy alone is indicated. If the patient has daily headaches, daily abortive agents should not be used and a preventative medication should be initiated. In addition neurologic work-up is higher priority in a patient with daily headache than in a patient with migraine.

Patients with migraines may, of course, get other diseases. Migraines rarely last for more than 48 hours, so the presence of headache for days suggests an alternative diagnosis. She most likely has cryptococcal meningitis. Before the era of AIDS cryptococcal meningitis was seen only occasionally. The incidence has increased

greatly since the spread of HIV. Treatment of cryptococcal meningitis in AIDS patients is different than in patients without AIDS, but
this will not be covered here as such patients would be referred for
urgent hospital admission..

Multiple sclerosis

Presentation

A 36-year-old man presents with diplopia. He has been seeing double
for approximately two weeks. The symptoms are getting slightly better
but still interfere with his reading and fine work. There were no
precipitating factors. This has never happened before, although on
detailed questioning, he did report that 5 years ago he temporarily
lost vision in his right eye. The vision returned over the ensuing 8
weeks. Also, 6 years prior to that episode he was diagnosed with the
'flu' and was unable to get out of bed for two weeks due to leg
weakness. He recalls little back pain and no fever, but gradually
improved without specific treatment.

The exam shows impaired adduction of the right eye with left gaze.
Other eye movements are normal, and he has a tendency to keep
his head turned slightly to the right to minimize the diplopia. Also,
he had bilateral upgoing plantar responses (Babinski signs).

The internuclear ophthalmoplegia along with the history of previous temporary neurological deficits raises concern about multiple
sclerosis.

Diagnosis

Referral to the neurologist results in the eventual diagnosis of multiple sclerosis on the basis of MRI findings, evoked potential findings,
and abnormal cerebrospinal fluid. MRI showed multiple areas of
increased signal intensity on T2-weighted images. Evoked potentials
showed not only optic nerve abnormalities but also a delay in
conduction through the thoracic spinal cord. CSF shows oligoclonal
bands in the CSF only (not blood) and high IgG index.

Management

Methylprednisolone 1 g daily i.v. is administered for 5 days. At the same time, the patient is begun on interferon β1A and does well. Continued physical therapy is ordered and medical supplies are ordered for the home.

Clinical course

Two years later, he then has an episode of weakness in the right leg which then begins to affect the left leg. Methylprednisolone is administered intravenously at 1 g/day for 5 days. With time and physical therapy the patient improves and he is allowed ultimately to return to work.

Discussion

The diagnosis of multiple sclerosis is obvious in this patient. The episode of leg weakness that was attributed to the flu was probably an episode of transverse myelitis. Most patients with transverse myelitis or optic neuritis do not go on to develop multiple sclerosis, but some do, so the patients should not be reassured that this kind of deficit could not recur.

Imaging with MRI is essential to diagnosis of MS. One can debate the requirements for evoked potentials and CSF sampling, but without the MRI, the diagnosis is always in doubt. The MRI is not always definitive, as there are other conditions that may produce similar appearances on the MRI. Multiple infarctions is the main diagnosis which needs to be eliminated by MRI and other testing.

Most patients with relapsing remitting MS should be placed on interferons or copaxone. These drugs reduce the rate of lesion accumulation by about 20% per year.

Appendix

Treatment of common neurologic disorders

See Table A.1.

Questionnaires

The following questionnaires have been developed as part of our clinical practice. The patient is typically given the questionnaire when first reporting a complaint. If the problem is chronic and does not seem serious, the questionnaire can be filled out by the patient before the next visit. Even a new or emergency patient may often be facilitated by having the patient fill in the questionnaire while they are waiting.

Table A.1 Treatment of common neurological disorders

Disorder	Treatment
Dementia – Alzheimer's – behavior	Cholinesterase inhibitors, risperidone, thioridazine, lorazepam
Dementia – Alzheimer's – cognition	Donepezil, rivastigmine, galantamine
Dementia – Parkinsonism – behavior	Olanzapine, quetiapine, thioridazine, clozapine
Dementia – Parkinsonism – cognition	Donepezil, rivastigmine, galantamine
Dementia – vascular – cognition	Pentoxyphylline, ergoloid mesylates (USA)
Headache – cluster – abortive treatment	Sumatriptan, oxygen
Headache – cluster – prevention	Prednisolone, verapamil
Headache – migraine – abortive treatment	Triptans, pure analgesics, combinations including butabital-containing and isomethaptine-containing agents
Headache – migraine – prevention	Amitriptyline, verapamil, valproate, gabapentin, propranolol
Myoclonus	Valproate, clonazepam, leveitracetam
Orthostatic hypotension	Fludrocortisone, midodrine (USA), high-salt diet
Pain – neuropathic – large fiber	Carbamazepine, gabapentin, oxcarbazepine
Pain – neuropathic – small fiber	Amitriptyline, gabapentin, oxcarbazepine
Pain – trigeminal neuralgia	Carbamazepine, oxcarbazepine, gabapentin, baclofen
Pain – post-herpetic neuralgia	Amitriptyline, carbamazepine, gabapentin
Parkinsonism – rigidity and bradykinesia	Levodopa, amantadine, ropinerole, pramipexole
Parkinsonism – tremor	Trihexyphenidyl, levodopa
Seizures – generalized – absence	Ethosuximide, lamotrigine, valproate
Seizures – generalized tonic-clonic	Phenytoin, carbamazepine, valproate
Seizures – partial – complex	Carbamazepine, oxcarbazepine, phenytoin, levetiracetam, zonisamide (USA), gabapentin
Seizures – partial – simple	Phenytoin, carbamazepine
Vertigo	Betahistine, promethazine

HEADACHE

Name:_____

Date:_____

Do you have different types of headache? If so, anwer these questions for each.

Describe the pain as accurately as you can (e.g. aching, throbbing, sharp, burning, tightness etc.).

How severe is the pain?

How can you tell when the pain is going to start?

What do you do when the pain begins?

Does anything bring it on or make it worse?

Does anything ease the pain?

How often do you have the pain?

How long does it last?

Is it worse at any particular time(s) of the day, week or month?

When, approximately, and under what circumstances, did it first begin?

What was going on in your life at that time?

Please list any other symptoms you associate with the headache

Are you more depressed, worried or irritable than usual?

How is your sleep pattern? (including ease of dropping off, wakening in the early hours and comment on sleep quality)

What are your smoking and drinking habits?

Please express any views, opinions, theories or fears which may have been suggested or crossed your mind as the cause of your symptoms

Is there anything else I should know?

Now please draw on the diagrams where the pain starts and mark how it spreads or moves

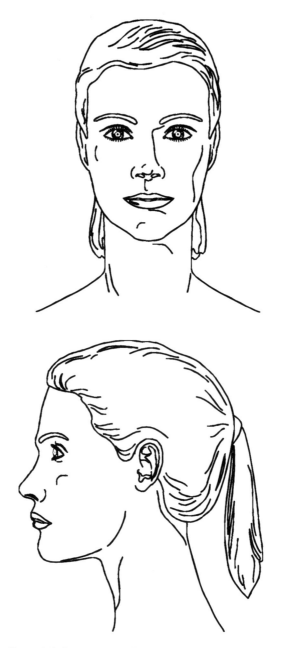

Figure A.1 *Face diagrams for the headache questionnaire.*

DIZZINESS

Name:_____

Date:_____

Describe the 'dizziness' as accurately as you can.

When, approximately, and under what circumstances, did it first begin?

What was going on in your life at that time?

Does anything bring it on or make it worse?

Does anything make it better?

How often do you get 'dizziness'?

How long does it last?

Is it worse at any particular time(s) of the day, week or month?

Please list any other symptoms you associate with the dizziness

Are you more depressed, worried or irritable than usual?

How is your sleep pattern? (including ease of dropping off, wakening in the early hours and comment on sleep quality)

What are your smoking and drinking habits?

Please express any views, opinions, theories or fears which may have been suggested or crossed your mind as the cause of your symptoms

Is there anything else I should know?

WEAKNESS AND FATIGUE

Name: _____

Today's date:_____

Describe your problem as accurately as you can

When, approximately, did it first begin?

What was going on in your life at that time?

Does it vary as the day or week goes on?

Does it vary with your menstrual cycle?

Please list any other symptoms you associate with the tiredness

Do you have any pain? If so, where and what pattern?

How is your sleep pattern? (including ease of dropping off, wakening in the early hours and does it refresh and restore you?)

Are you gaining or losing weight?

Are you more depressed, worried or irritable than normal?

What are your smoking and drinking habits?

Is your job easy or demanding?

Could anything in your lifestyle be making your symptom worse?

Please express any views, opinions, theories or fears which may have been suggested or crossed your mind as the cause of your symptoms

Is there anything else I should know?

SEIZURES AND OTHER SPELLS

Name:_____

Today's date:_____

Tell me about your spells with as much detail as possible.

For a single spell, or your last spell:

> When did it occur?
> How long did it last?
> What exactly happened during that spell?
> Did you become unconscious?
> Did you lose control of your bladder or bowels?
> How did observers describe your spell?
> How did you feel after a spell? Were you sick, confused, drowsy or feel fine?

If you have had multiple spells:

> When did they start?
> How many have you had?
> How often do they occur?
> When was the last spell?

Do you have any warning that you are about to have a spell?

What seems to trigger a spell?

Do you drink alcohol? How much and how often?

Have any tests been done so far?

What are you concerned about? Do you suspect or fear any specific diagnosis?

Is there anything else I should know about the spells?

Patient handouts

Attached are patient handouts on a variety of common neurological disorders.

Some of the most reliable internet sites for information are:

- US National Library of Medicine for patients: www.medlineplus.gov
- American Academy of Neurology. Has on-line versions of patient information brochures: www.aan.com
- Mayo Clinic information service: www.mayoclinic.com

DEMENTIA

What is dementia?

Dementia means loss of memory and problem-solving ability. This is a common condition and increases in likelihood with age. Currently, more than 10 million Americans have dementia.

The most common causes of dementia are:

- Alzheimer's disease
- Multiple strokes
- Other degenerative dementias
- Problems with metabolism
- Hydrocephalus (fluid on the brain)
- Effects of medicines
- Depression

Alzheimer's disease is the most common cause of dementia, responsible for about half of cases. Patients have loss of memory and other cognitive processes. The cause is thought to be a combination of genetic factors with perhaps some contribution from the environment. Multiple strokes produces vascular dementia, which means that there is damage to the blood vessels. Vascular dementia is more common in patients with high blood pressure, diabetes, high cholesterol, and in those who smoke. Other degenerative dementias include some patients with symptoms of Parkinson's disease who also have memory loss as well as other conditions which produce loss of function of the nerve cells. Medicines commonly produce confusion, and you would be hard-pressed to find some that did not have the potential to produce confusion, dizziness, or nausea. Nevertheless, we need to consider current medicines in every person who complains of memory loss. Depression affects attention and concentration, so this is considered a potential cause for dementia, when in reality, it is not dementia at all. Problems with metabolism include thyroid hormone deficiency, vitamin B12 deficiency, and a few others. Hydrocephalus is excess fluid in the skull. This can be due to two causes: too much fluid is made or the fluid is not draining adequately. The latter is by far the most common.

How is dementia diagnosed?

Dementia is a clinical diagnosis. This means that the diagnosis is made on the basis of history and exam findings. Tests usually done in patients with dementia include:

- CT or MRI of the brain
- Lab tests including chemistries, blood count, thyroid function tests, and test of some vitamin levels

Sometimes, other tests are done, including psychological testing, other types of scans, or additional blood work. Rarely, a sample of spinal fluid may have to be obtained by spinal tap. On the basis of these tests, one of the diagnoses listed above can be identified.

How is dementia treated?

Treatment totally depends on the cause. The most research has been done on patients with Alzheimer's disease and other degenerative dementias. There are several medicines which are used for this including:

- donepezil (Aricept)
- galantamine (Reminyl)
- rivastigmine (Exelon)
- tacrine (Cognex).

Different patients respond to different medicines, so if one does not work or is not tolerated, one of the others should be used.

Sometimes, medicines are needed to treat anxiety, depression, or fear and anger. These emotions are common in patients with dementia, especially. The medicines used for these symptoms are the same ones used for patients with these emotions who do not have dementia.

People with vascular dementia may respond to these medicines, but this is still under experimental study. Much more important is prevention of further strokes, which can allow the healing process to occur. Therefore, treatment of hypertension, diabetes, high cholesterol, and smoking can be helpful. Depression is treated with one of many available agents. Patients with depression often have more of an improvement in memory than patients with other causes of memory loss. Hydrocephalus can improve with drainage of the fluid, but this is a surgical procedure with the potential for complications. Also, drainage of the fluid gives the person the chance to improve, but does not guarantee improvement.

What can be expected?

Presently, there is no cure for most patients with dementia. The medicines can improve memory and emotions for as long as the medicines are given. Scientists are working on medicines and other treatments which would actually fix the loss of nerve cells, but these treatments are unproved and still experimental.

What can I do to help myself?

Most physicians recommend taking some nutritional supplements to try to stem the progression of some types of dementia, especially Alzheimer's disease and other degenerative dementias. While there is not a lot of scientific evidence for this, we often recommend the following:

- vitamin E 1000 IU/day
- vitamin C 250 mg/day
- ibuprofen or similar anti-inflammatory medicine.

Scientific studies indicate that remaining intellectually active has a protective effect on preventing some kinds of dementia, especially Alzheimer's disease. We do not want to do mental gymnastics to the point of becoming frustrated, but maintaining active interests appears to be helpful.

Where can I get additional information?

- Alzheimer's Association: www.alz.org or phone 800-272-3900
- National Library of Medicine Information on Memory Loss and Dementia: www.nlm.nih.gov/medlineplus/dementia.html
- National Library of Medicine Information on Alzheimer's Disease: www.nlm.nih.gov/medlineplus/alzheimersdisease.html

ESSENTIAL TREMOR

What is essential tremor?

Essential tremor is the most common cause of tremor seen in medical practice. The tremor is present usually in the arms but may also involve the head. At rest, the arms and hands are still, but with activity there is shaking. Fatigue and nervousness tend to worsen the tremor.

Essential tremor tends to be familial. The onset is often in middle age or senior years, although essential tremor can even be seen in children.

The exact cause of essential tremor is unknown but it is thought to be an imbalance in how the circuits of the brain control movement. There is nothing that someone does to make them more likely to develop the tremor. Essential tremor does not lead into Parkinson's disease or other diseases.

How is essential tremor diagnosed?

Essential tremor is a clinical diagnosis. This means that the diagnosis is based on the combination of history and exam findings during the clinic visit. There are no scans or lab tests which make the diagnosis. If there are some unusual features of the tremor noticed by the physician, then some tests may be ordered. The possible tests which may be ordered include a scan and tests of thyroid function, but others may be recommended.

How is essential tremor treated?

There are several medicines which can help essential tremor, but not all patients need to be treated. If the tremor is mild, the person may decide to forego treatment until it becomes worse.

If treatment is needed, the following medicines are mainly used:

- propranolol (Inderal)
- primidone (Mysoline)
- gabapentin (Neurontin)
- topiramate (Topamax)
- clonazepam (USA: Klonopin, UK: Rivotril)

There are a few other medicines which are occasionally used, but these are the most commonly used.

Surgical treatment is offered for the rare patient who has very disabling tremor which does not respond to medical treatment. However, there are real risks associated with surgery, and it is not a cure, so surgery is not a viable option for most people.

What can be expected?

Presently, there is no cure for essential tremor. The medicines can improve the tremor but do not totally abolish it.

Luckily, essential tremor does not interfere with normal life for most people. Some people have tremor severe enough to interfere with fine manual activities, but they are still able to carry out full and productive lives.

What can I do to help myself?

There are only a few things people can do to reduce the tremor. Some of these include:

- reduce caffeine intake;
- get adequate rest;
- low alcohol intake;
- quit smoking;
- have arms supported during fine manipulations.

While none of these will cure the tremor, they can minimize the tremor.

Sources for additional information:

- Parkinson's Institute tremor page:
  www.parkinsonsinstitute.org/tremor.html
- International Tremor Foundation: www.essentialtremor.org
- More detailed info from eMedicine:
  www.emedicine.com/neuro/topic129.htm

MIGRAINE

What is migraine?

Migraine is one of the most common causes of headache. The cause is thought to be inflammation of the blood vessels of the scalp. Therefore, this is sometimes referred to as a *vascular headache.*

What causes migraine?

Migraine occurs in some people because they have a genetic predisposition. About 80% of patients with migraine have a family history of migraine or other vascular headache. Migraine is more likely to develop in people with certain hormonal changes, including during the menses and near the time of menopause.

How is migraine diagnosed?

Migraine is a clinical diagnosis. This means that the combination of history and exam makes the diagnosis; there are no tests which can show migraine. On the other hand, tests are sometimes performed to look for other conditions.

When headaches occur off-and-on, the chance of finding some serious abnormality on laboratory test is extremely low. If someone does not respond to treatment, a CT or MRI may be performed, but usually this is normal.

How is a migraine treated?

There are many medications which are used for migraine. The most common of these are of two basic types: triptans and pain relievers. *Triptans* is the name for a class of drugs which include Imigran

(USA: Imitrex), Maxalt, Zomig, and Amerge. There are others in the group which should be available in the future.

Pain relievers include Tylenol, aspirin, and prescription drugs. Many of these contain caffeine, which has some beneficial effect on migraine by itself.

We try to avoid pain relievers for migraine because the triptans are usually more effective and can allow the patient to return to work or school quite quickly. The pain relievers can, unfortunately, cause a rebound headache. This is where a dose of pain medicine is followed by a recurrence of headache later that day or the following day. A vicious cycle is created which eventually results in the patient having to take pain medicine every day. This is one of the most common causes of headache, and can only be treated by stopping the use of all pain medicines.

How can migraine be prevented?

Migraine cannot usually be totally prevented, but can be controlled in most instances, reducing the incidence to acceptable levels.

Self-help measures can significantly reduce the incidence of migraine attacks. Some of these suggestions are presented at the end of this sheet.

Preventatives are usually given when someone has a migraine at least four times in a month. Less frequent headaches do not warrant daily medication except in certain circumstances. Some of the preventative medicines are:

- cyproheptadine (Periactin)
- gabapentin (Neurontin)
- oxcarbazepine (Trileptal)
- propranolol (Inderal)
- topiramate (Topamax)
- valproate (UK: Epilim; USA: Depakote)
- verapamil (various)

These are in alphabetical order, and not in the order that they would be used. To a certain extent, the medicines used are dependent on the patient's medical details, but it is also an element of trial-and-error. If one medicine does not work, then another is tried.

Preventative medicines cannot stop all headaches. They reduce the number of headaches for most patients, and may also shorten them.

What can be expected?

Migraine can be improved in most people. Medicines plus following self-help guidelines reduce the frequency of headaches and shorten attacks when they do occur. Therefore, most people have improvement in their headaches. Unfortunately, the medicines cannot stop or prevent every headache, and cannot stop all headaches.

Migraines usually get less frequent and less severe with age. They often stop somewhere between 35 and 50 years of age. While some people have migraines after these ages, this is uncommon.

During a migraine, your head might feel like it is going to explode, but of course, this never happens. It may seem as if a headache this bad has to indicate a severe problem with the brain, but luckily, this is not the case. Eventually, the headache will go away.

What can I do to help myself?

There are a few suggestions which can reduce the number of migraines.

- sleep regularly
- eat a balanced diet
- keep body weight normal
- avoid chemicals which trigger headaches
- avoid taking pain medicines frequently
- exercise regularly.

Exercise can help to improve headache frequency, and it should be done three times per week for at least 40 minutes at a time. Diabetics should have a different schedule, perhaps exercising 15 minutes twice daily.

Certain foods can trigger migraines in some people. These are not important for all people, but you might try to avoid the following to reduce the number of headaches:

- *MSG – monosodium glutamate:* typically found in prepared foods, not just Chinese food. Even pizza and barbecue may have MSG.
- *Aspartame – Nutrasweet:* in most diet drinks. Reported to trigger migraines in some people.
- *Nitrates and nitrites:* found in some packaged meats.
- *Sharp cheeses:* a factor for a small number of patients.
- *Red wines:* may cause a headache not just when consumed but also the next day.
- *Chocolate:* a factor for a small number of patients.

Caffeine deserves special comment. High doses of caffeine can cause headaches in some people. More common is caffeine-withdrawal headache, however. This happens when someone misses their morning or afternoon caffeine-containing drink.

Pain medicines are frequently used for patients with migraine, and there are a few over-the-counter medicines. However, it is important to remember that too many pain medicines can produce rebound headache.

More information

- JAMA migraine info page: www.ama-assn.org/special/migraine/migraine.htm
- NIH: www.nlm.nih.gov/medlineplus/headacheandmigraine.html

MULTIPLE SCLEROSIS

What is multiple sclerosis?

Multiple sclerosis (MS) is a neurological condition which produces areas of inflammation and damage in the white matter of the brain. The white matter is composed of connecting tissues; essentially the wires connecting the different parts of the brain.

The cause of MS is not known, but there is a problem with the immune system in that it attacks your own nerves. More precisely, the immune system attacks the insulation of the nerve cells, called the myelin sheath. Therefore, MS is sometimes called a *demyelinating disease*, since the myelin is damaged.

MS may be caused by an infection, although the details are not completely known. When we get an infection, our immune system attacks the virus or bacterium, usually killing it. However, once in a while, the immune attack turns against the person's own body, thereby causing diseases. In some people, this causes a single attack which is like MS but only happens once. In some people, the immune system produces repeated attacks, and this is MS.

How is multiple sclerosis diagnosed?

MS is diagnosed by a combination of symptoms, findings on exam, and lab tests. The most important lab test is MRI. This test is able to show the areas of inflammation in almost all patients with MS. Lumbar puncture (LP) is occasionally done; this is also called a spinal tap. The spinal fluid tests are compared to blood tests to support the diagnosis of MS.

The diagnosis of MS may not be able to be made with certainty in mild cases or very early in the disease. Repeated evaluation in the clinic and with additional tests may be needed to cinch the diagnosis.

How is multiple sclerosis treated?

There are several kinds of treatments. These include:

- protective treatment
- abortive treatment
- fatigue treatment
- spasticity treatment.

Protective treatments. Beta-interferons help to reduce the chance of MS attacks, and reduce ensuing disability. At present there are three preparations of beta-interferon on the market; they are all given by injection. These drugs do not prevent 100% of attacks, so having an occasional attack does not mean that the drug is not working.

Abortive treatment with Solu-Medrone is used for acute attacks in most patients. This is given intravenously for 3 to 7 days, depending on the individual situation. While Solu-Medrone shortens the duration of an attack, it does not change the amount of recovery which will occur, so there is not a problem if someone cannot tolerate or get the infusions.

Fatigue is a common problem in patients with MS. We are not as good as we would like to be in improving fatigue. Two medicines are mainly used for this: amantadine and provigil. Amantadine is a drug which was developed as an antiviral drug, but has been found to help fatigue in some patients with MS. Provigil was developed for patients with narcolepsy – a condition where there are sleep attacks. Recent research has found that this can be helpful for some patients with MS.

Spasticity is muscle stiffness which develops in many people with MS. Medicines for this include baclofen, zanaflex, valium, and dantrium. Patients respond differently, so more than one of these may have to be tried.

Novantrone is a chemotherapeutic drug which has recently been found to reduce the rate of worsening in patients with an uncommon progressive form of MS. Unfortunately, Novantrone helps for 2–3 years, and does not cure the disease. Therefore, this drug is not appropriate for most patients with MS.

Depression is common in patients with MS. While most patients eventually adapt to having a chronic condition without use of medicines, we do not hesitate to use medicines for depression if needed. Depression may not be noticed in the clinic, so if the patient or family members notice symptoms of depression, they should be discussed with the doctor.

New research is constantly being done. Antibiotics are given to some patients because of the theory that some bacteria may produce the changes to the immune system which causes MS. Also, medicines are currently under development which may be able to improve the functioning of damaged nerve cells. So far, these studies are very preliminary, and they may or may not be eventually found to be helpful.

What can be expected?

MS is usually associated with relapses and remissions. This means that there are periodic worsenings and improvements. Treatments can shorten worsenings and decrease the frequency of worsenings, but cannot totally prevent them. Therefore, most patients have occasional attacks, but we try to minimize the attacks and minimize the disability produced by each.

What can I do to help myself?

Nothing that the person did during their life caused MS. We know of no way we can avoid getting it. However, when one has MS, there are a few simple guidelines which should be followed:

- See your doctor regularly and especially contact your doctor if you have an attack.
- Get plenty of rest.
- Maintain normal activity and even job, as much as possible.
- Avoid getting overheated, since this can worsen the function of damaged nerve cells.

In addition, the person with MS should consider joining support groups and getting on the mailing lists of national MS organizations. As with all chronic conditions, a personal adaptation to the condition is essential. This is more easily said than done. Family support, medical information, and sometimes even counseling may be needed.

PARKINSON'S DISEASE

What is Parkinson's disease?

Parkinson's disease is a condition which produces slowness and stiffness of muscles, often with tremor of the arms. Other symptoms include loss of balance and inability to make fine movements of the hands.

The symptoms of Parkinson's disease are due to damage to the centers which control movement deep in the brain. For most people, the cause of Parkinson's disease is unknown. Years ago, some patients would develop Parkinson's disease after a viral infection of the brain or after taking in some toxic chemicals, but this is rare now. Occasionally, symptoms of Parkinson's disease can develop when certain nerve medicines are given, but fortunately, this improves when the medicine is stopped. Small strokes can also produce the symptoms of Parkinson's disease.

How is Parkinson's diagnosed?

Parkinson's disease is a clinical diagnosis. This means that the diagnosis is made on the basis of history and exam findings. Tests are usually done to look for other causes of muscle stiffness, imbalance, and tremor and they essentially rule out other causes. Tests usually done in patients with suspected Parkinson's disease include:

- CT or MRI of the brain;
- lab tests including chemistries, blood count, thyroid function tests, and test of some vitamin levels

There are occasionally other tests which are performed, but these are the most important.

How is Parkinson's treated?

There are several types of medicines which can help Parkinson's disease. These are divided into classes which help the doctor select the right types of drug for each patient. The functions of the classes are as follows:

- Decrease effects of acetylcholine in the brain.
- Make more dopamine.
- Stimulate the dopamine receptor.
- Increase release of dopamine from the brain cells.
- Block the breakdown of dopamine, leaving more available for the brain.

All of these medicines either increase level of effect of dopamine in the brain or decrease the effect of acetylcholine on the brain. Increasing dopamine improves muscle stiffness and ease of movement, including walking. Decreasing acetylcholine reduces tremor. Therefore, the particular drug used depends partly on which is the most prominent symptoms – tremor or stiffness.

In these types, there are several medicines: some of the important ones and their type are:

- Artane (decreases acetylcholine in the brain);
- Sinemet (makes more dopamine);
- Symmetrel (stimulates release of dopamine);
- Requip (stimulates dopamine receptor);
- Mirapex (stimulates dopamine receptor);
- Eldepryl (prevents breakdown of dopamine);
- Comtan (prevents breakdown of dopamine).

Artane and other drugs which block the effect of acetylcholine mainly benefit tremor. There is no definite benefit on muscle stiffness and movement.

Sinemet increases the production of dopamine, and helps muscle stiffness and slowness of movement. There is some improvement in tremor, but less so than with Artane.

Requip and *Mirapex* directly stimulate the dopamine receptor and both can help movements and stiffness.

Amantadine increases the release of dopamine from the nerves of the brain. This can be mildly helpful for patients with muscle stiffness and tremor, but has a weaker effect than the other listed drugs. Amantadine can reduce extra flapping movements which can develop with the other medicines, however.

Eldepryl and *Comtan* decrease the breakdown of dopamine, thereby increasing the effect of dopamine on the brain. They work through very different mechanisms and have different uses. Comtan is always used with Sinemet, since it increases the duration of benefit of Sinemet rather than having its own direct effect on Parkinson's disease.

Surgery is being performed in some universities for Parkinson's disease. This should still be considered experimental since the exact methods are still being researched. However, surgery can be of help especially for the tremor of Parkinson's disease. It is important to realize that surgery is not a cure, and most patients will continue to have significant symptoms after surgery.

What can be expected?

Currently, there is no cure for Parkinson's disease. Over time, the symptoms gradually get worse. Medicines can make the symptoms better, but they do not prevent eventual worsening. Nevertheless, the condition gets worse slowly, so that most patients have years of good function.

What can I do to help myself?

Most physicians recommend taking some nutritional supplements to try to stem the progression of Parkinson's disease. While there is not a lot of scientific evidence for this, we often recommend the following:

- Vitamin E 1000 IU/day
- Vitamin C 250 mg/day
- Multivitamin daily.

These cannot prevent the progression of the condition, but the chance of side-effects is low and there is some potential for clinical stabilization.

Additional information

- NIH Health Information:
  www.nlm.nih.gov/medlineplus/parkinsonsdisease.html
- Parkinson's Disease Foundation: www.pdf.org
- American Parkinson's Disease Association: www.apdaparkinson.com

PERIPHERAL NEUROPATHY

What is neuropathy?

Neuropathy is damage to one or more nerves in the body. The nerve damage can cause numbness, pain, and weakness. The location of the symptoms depends on the location of the damage. Some of the most common forms of neuropathy are:

- Peripheral neuropathy
- Carpal tunnel syndrome
- Ulnar neuropathy
- Peroneal neuropathy.

Peripheral neuropathy is where the damage is to multiple nerves in the body. The longest nerves are mainly affected, such that the hands and feet develop symptoms before other areas. The most common cause of peripheral neuropathy is diabetes, although there are many other possible causes which should be looked for.

Carpal tunnel syndrome is damage to the median nerve at the wrist. This is a large nerve which passes through the palm. Carpal tunnel syndrome produces numbness on the palm of the hand and frequently also produces pain at the wrist. The cause is usually a combination of individual anatomy of the carpal tunnel plus repetitive activity of the wrist. Most patients notice that the symptoms are most prominent with repetitive motion of the wrist, with tight grip on an object such as a steering wheel, and at night, when increased fluid in the arm and odd postures can aggravate carpal tunnel syndrome.

Ulnar neuropathy produces numbness on part of the palm of the hand and pain in the forearm or elbow. This is usually due to damage to the ulnar nerve as it crosses the elbow (the 'funny bone') or down in the forearm. Repetitive stretch or injury to the ulnar nerve is usually responsible for the damage. Patients with diabetes are especially likely to develop this.

Peroneal neuropathy produces weakness of lifting the foot along with numbness on the top of the foot.

How is neuropathy diagnosed?

Neuropathy is suspected from symptoms and findings on exam. The EMG confirms the diagnosis for most people, although a few patients will not have abnormal EMG.

EMG stands for *electromyogram*. This is a test of the muscles and nerves which involves two parts. The first part is stimulation of the nerves with a very brief electrical pulse while we record from the nerves and muscles. The second part involves placing a small needle into the muscles. The needle has a tiny electrode at the tip which records the electricity coming from the muscles. The EMG can tell what type of nerve or muscle damage is present and predict what the likely cause is, but since different causes of nerve and muscle damage can cause similar findings on EMG, additional blood tests are usually needed.

Blood tests can look for common causes of nerve and muscle damage, although in some people, we cannot determine a definite cause. Which blood tests are done depends on the patient's neuropathy, but usually thyroid tests and measures of some vitamin levels such as B12 are commonly performed. Other blood tests and urine tests may be needed.

How is neuropathy treated?

If we can find a cause for the neuropathy, then a treatment may be able to cure it. Unfortunately, some types of neuropathy are incurable. If we do not determine a cause for the neuropathy, then it is also essentially incurable. Scientists are working on medicines to make damaged nerves grow, but no medicine has been proven effective yet.

While we cannot cure neuropathy in many people, we can usually improve the symptoms. Many people with neuropathy have unpleasant sensations in the area of damage. These symptoms may include burning pain, shooting pain, tingling, and numbness. Numbness is decreased feeling. All of these symptoms except numbness can be helped by medicines. Some of the medicines are:

- gabapentin
- amitriptyline
- carbamazepine
- oxcarbazepine
- lamotrigine.

This is just a few of the drugs which we use for neuropathy; there are others which are sometimes used. Which medicine to use depends on the particular condition, but is partly trial-and-error. This means that different medicines are tried until one is found which works.

What can be expected?

Neuropathy is a common condition, afflicting millions of people in the USA. Fortunately, it is rare for neuropathy to put someone in a wheelchair. Neuropathy is not a fatal illness. In addition, most people with neuropathy have pain for a few months or years then the pain goes away, even though the cause could not be reversed. This is because damaged nerves cause pain, but when the nerves stop working altogether, the pain goes away. Numbness persists, but at least the pain is relieved.

What can I do to help myself?

To reduce the damage to the nerves, we need to take as best care of ourselves as possible. We recommend:

- balanced diet
- vitamin supplements
- exercise
- avoid alcohol
- if diabetic – be especially good about controlling glucose.

Vitamins have not been proven to improve neuropathy if a vitamin deficiency is not identified, but most doctors recommend taking a multivitamin daily. Extra B12, C, and E are also taken by many people with neuropathy.

Additional information

- Good book for patients: www.medpress.com/index.html
- NIH: www.ninds.nih.gov/health_and_medical/disorders/ peripheralneuropathy_doc.htm
- More detailed info: www.aafp.org/afp/980215ap/poncelet.html

STROKE AND TIA

What is stroke?

Stroke is damage to the brain due to a problem with the blood vessels. The most common type is blockage of an artery. Other types include breakage of an artery and blockage of a vein. People with stroke can have a wide variety of symptoms, including paralysis of one part of the body, loss of speech or swallowing, loss of vision, imbalance, and even unconsciousness. The symptoms depend on which blood vessels are damaged.

What is a TIA?

TIA stands for transient ischemic attack. This means that there is blockage of an artery, as with a stroke, but the blockage is only temporary, so the blood supply to the brain is returned and any damage is repaired. All of the symptoms of a stroke can develop, but the symptoms are temporary. TIA is sometimes called 'ministroke' but this is not a medical term.

How are stroke and TIA diagnosed?

Stroke and TIA are clinical diagnoses. This means that the symptoms reported by the patient and the findings on exam make the diagnosis. No test can show a TIA. A CT or MRI can show a stroke, but even these tests often do not show the damage immediately.

What tests are needed?

Patients with TIA and stroke all have a scan, either *CT* or *MRI*. Which one to be done depends on the details of the patient's medical condition. This can make sure that there are not other causes of the symptoms other than stroke, such as tumor, infection, or multiple sclerosis.

Ultrasounds of the carotid arteries and heart are usually done to look for blockage of the arteries which might need surgery or damage to the heart which can make stroke and TIA more likely.

Blood tests are done to look especially for damage to liver, kidneys, and bone marrow which might alter treatment.

ECG is usually done to look for heart damage which can occur at the time of a stroke. *Chest x-ray* is usually done, especially in patients who smoke, to screen for tumors which also can make stroke more likely.

How are stroke and TIA treated?

There are two basic ways that stroke are treated. First, if someone has a stroke, we want to improve the blood supply to the damaged brain. Second, we want to reduce the chance of another stroke.

Restoring blood flow to the brain is best accomplished by blood-clot busters such as TPA (tissue plasminogen activator). Unfortunately, most stroke patients are not able to get TPA because they arrive too late for the medicine to be given. TPA has to be given within 3 hours from when the symptoms first began. If someone wakes up with a stroke, we do not know when the stroke started, and it is too danger-ous to give the medicine more than 3 hours after onset. In addition, there are a number of details about the patient's medical condition which would make us unable to give the TPA.

Blood thinners reduce the chance of recurrent stroke, but do not dissolve blockage that has already developed. This is important, though, since after having a TIA or stroke, the risk of having another makes it important to use these medicines. Some of the commonly used blood thinners are:

- aspirin
- warfarin
- heparin

- persantine
- plavix
- ticlid.

Which drug to use depends on the details of the patient's condition. Aspirin is most commonly used.

If a stroke leaves a patient with weakness, therapy may be needed to improve function. Physical therapy helps actual movements. Occupational therapy helps patients do things for themselves. Speech therapy helps speech and swallowing. If the weakness is severe enough, stay in a rehab unit can be of tremendous help.

What can be expected?

Most patients with stroke improve, although the improvement varies between patients. Some patients improve to almost normal, others are totally dependent on others. Most are somewhere in between.

Attitude is tremendously important. As we go through life, we can either be happy for our abilities and gifts or we can resent what we do not have. This is especially true after a stroke. If we are slightly impatient and grasp onto every improvement, we can be pleased with our life after stroke. If not, we can become bitter and this can even slow recovery. The father of one of the Semmes–Murphey doctors had a massive stroke which left him paralyzed on the left side, depending on a wheelchair, but still able to live at home. After about two months of rehab, he summarized his condition, 'I wish I would have improved more, but I can be happy like I am'. If we can seize this attitude, we can live a better life even after a devastating event like a stroke.

What can I do to help myself?

The best treatment of a stroke is prevention. After a TIA or stroke, most people are pretty good about taking medicines and improving life style to prevent another stroke. However, we should not wait until after the first stroke or TIA – the first stroke may kill us. To reduce the chance of stroke, we should do the following:

- check and control blood pressure;
- check and control cholesterol;
- not smoke;
- not drink alcohol to excess;
- eat a balanced, low-fat diet;
- keep weight where it should be;
- take blood thinners if we have already had a TIA or stroke.

None of us are perfect about this, even doctors. But if we could just do a little better, we could reduce the chance of stroke and death tremendously.

SEIZURES AND EPILEPSY

What are seizures?

Seizures are episodes where there is an abnormal pattern of electricity in the brain. The entire brain may be affected or only part of the brain. The symptoms of seizures differ markedly between people, and may differ between seizures in a single patient. Some of the possible seizure types are:

- *Generalized tonic-clonic:* the person becomes unconsciousness and shakes or stiffens the arms and legs.
- *Absence:* the person (usually a child) stops moving or speaking and stares without any shaking of stiffening.
- *Simple partial:* the person may shake one arm uncontrollably, after which they cannot move it.
- *Complex partial:* the person cannot respond but remains seated or standing and may have smacking movements of the lips or some other repetitive activity.

There are other seizure types, but the ones listed are the most common. There are some important things to remember about what are **not** seizures. Some people will have spells which may look like seizures, but the physician can tell by either history or examination or tests that the episodes are not true seizures; they can be triggered by nerves. Also, some patients can black-out because of lack of circulation to the brain. This can produce some twitching of the limbs when the person is unconscious, but is due to lack of oxygen, and not a seizure, as such. Lastly, aggressive outbursts and violence directed against someone is not a seizure.

There are many possible causes of seizures, including:

- inheritance
- head injury
- alcohol and drugs
- infections

- stroke
- developmental abnormalities.

Scar tissue can form from almost any brain problem, and this can cause seizures from weeks to months later. *Developmental abnormalities* include a number of variations in the way the nerve cells are connected. Some, but not all, of these are associated with changed physical appearance and/or learning difficulties.

What is epilepsy?

Epilepsy means recurrent **unprovoked** seizures. This means that someone who has seizures all associated with a defined cause, such as acute head injury or alcohol, does not have epilepsy. However, the damage to the nerve cells from this can produce epilepsy, such that the person has seizures even when unprovoked.

How are seizures diagnosed?

Seizures are usually diagnosed by the history from the patient and observers. EEG is almost always done, but does not show seizure activity in all patients unless done during a seizure.

A scan is usually done, such as CT or MRI. This is usually normal, although occasionally we may find small areas of scar tissue, cysts, or benign growths. While we will occasionally see malignant tumors, this is uncommon. Most people do **not** have tumors.

The diagnosis of seizure may be uncertain initially, especially when the symptoms and reports from observers do not seem to indicate clear seizure activity. Therefore, additional history from observers and repeated testing is occasionally needed. Sometimes, patients are admitted to the hospital for a few hours or even a day to record the brain activity continuously and to determine whether a spell is a seizure.

How are seizures treated?

Seizures are usually treated with medicines, although if someone has a single seizure, treatment is not always needed. Whether to treat depends on the person's clinical situation and results of the diagnostic tests. If treatment is needed, different medicines are used for different seizure types, alhough there are some overlaps between different seizure types. Among the medicines used for seizures are:

- valproate (Convulex)
- phenytoin (Dilantin)
- tiagabine (Gabitril)
- levetiracetam (Keppra)
- clonazepam (Rivotril)
- lamotrigine (Lamictal)
- primidone (Mysoline)
- gabapentin (Neurontin)
- phenobarbital (Phenobarbitone)
- carbamazepine (Tegretol)
- topiramate (Topamax)
- oxcarbazepine (Trileptal)
- ethosuximide (Zarontin)

More than one medicine may be needed for seizure control. If this is not effective in preventing seizures, there are some surgeries which can be done. Because of the risk of surgery, it is not done unless the patient has failed treatment with medicines. The most common surgery is removal of the seizure focus. Electrical stimulation of the vagus nerve with a pacemaker-like device is increasingly used, although this does not prevent all seizures.

What can be expected?

Seizures can be controlled in most patients. Some patients will still have occasional seizures, although the medicines reduce the number of seizures.

People with seizures worry about death from a seizure. Luckily, this is extremely rare. More common is death from having a seizure while driving. This is why patients who are having seizures should not drive until the doctor says it is safe. This is not just common sense – this is the law.

Seizures do not cause brain damage, so there should not be concern that every seizure is producing loss of brain function – it does not.

Children with seizures frequently grow out of them. However, about 30% will continue to have seizures later in life. Also, the chance of growing-out of seizures gets progressively less as the patient gets older.

What can I do to help myself?

We know that certain stresses on the body can make seizures worse, so minimizing these stresses can reduce the chance of seizures. In general, physical stress is more of a factor than mental stress – getting nervous is not likely to provoke an epileptic seizure, although it can provoke spells which look like seizures. Some of the best ways to take care of ourselves are:

- Eat right – have a balanced diet.
- Sleep well – get plenty of sleep.
- Don't drink alcohol – this increases the chance off seizures and affects the seizure medicines.
- Don't drive motor vehicles or do other dangerous activities if the seizures are not 100% controlled.

The doctor can give additional advice on activities, etc.

The most important thing a patient with seizures can do to minimize the chance of a seizure is to take the medicine correctly. Missing doses is the most common cause of a person with epilepsy having seizures despite being on medication.

Where can I get additional information?

- Epilepsy Foundation of America: www.efa.org
- National Library of Medicine:
  www.mln.nih.gov/medlineplus/epilepsy.html
- Epilepsy Research Foundation (UK): www.erf.org.uk
- British Epilepsy Association: www.epilepsy.org.uk or
  www.bea-connect.com Free helpline: 0808 800 5050

Index